Ultrasound Interactions in Biology and Medicine

Ultrasound Interactions in Biology and Medicine

Edited by

R. Millner, E. Rosenfeld, and U. Cobet

Institute of Applied Biophysics
Martin Luther University School of Medicine, Halle, German Democratic Republic

Plenum Press • New York and London

Library of Congress Cataloging in Publication Data

Main entry under title:

Ultrasound interactions in biology and medicine.

Includes bibliographical references and index.
"Proceedings of an International Symposium on Ultrasound Interaction in Biology and Medicine, held November 10–14, 1980, in Reinhardsbrunn, German Democratic Republic"—T.p. verso.
1. Ultrasonic waves—Physiological effect—Congresses. 2. Diagnosis, Ultrasonic —Congresses. 3. Ultrasonics in biology—Congresses. I. Millner, Rudolf. II. Rosenfeld, E. III. Cobet, U. IV. International Symposium on Ultrasound Interaction in Biology and Medicine (1980: Reinhardsbrunn, Germany) [DNLM: 1. Ultrasonics— Congresses. QC 244 I61u 1980]
QP82.2.U37U48 1983   616.07′543   83-9551
ISBN 978-1-4684-8386-4   ISBN 978-1-4684-8384-0 (eBook)
DOI 10.1007/978-1-4684-8384-0

Proceedings of an International Symposium on
Ultrasound Interaction in Biology and Medicine,
held November 10–14, 1980,
in Reinhardsbrunn, German Democratic Republic

© 1983 Plenum Press, New York
Softcover reprint of the hardcover 1st edition 1983
A Division of Plenum Publishing Corporation
233 Spring Street, New York, N.Y. 10013

SCIENTIFIC COMMITTEE:

Prof. Dr. R. Millner, Halle, GDR (Chairman)
Prof. Dr. L. Filipczynski, Warsaw, Poland
Prof. Dr. H. Hertz, Lund, Sweden
Doc. Dr. A.P. Sarvazyan, Puschino, USSR
Dr. C.R. Hill, Sutton, U.K.
Prof. Dr. J. Hrazdira, Brno, Czechoslovakia
Dr. N. Leitgeb, Graz, Austria

ORGANIZING COMMITTEE:

Dr. M. Koch, Berlin, GDR (Chairman)
A. Kollath, Berlin, GDR
Dr. E. Rosenfeld, Halle, GDR
Dr. U. Cobet, Halle, GDR
Dipl-Phys. A. Klemenz, Halle, GDR
Dipl-Phys. P. Schmidt, Halle, GDR

PREFACE

Due to the ever increasing interest in the use of non-invasive
ultrasonic methods in medical diagnostics on the one hand and the
specific effects of ultrasound in medical therapy on the other, the
questions of safety and optimal applications are topical and of great
importance.

For this reason the symposium "Ultrasound Interaction in Biology
and Medicine," initiated and supported by the "International
Organization of Medical Physics," took place. The organizers were
the Institute of Applied Biophysics of the Martin-Luther-University,
Halle (Saale), German Democratic Republic, in association with the
Society for Physical and Mathematical Biology of the GDR along with
other scientific organizations.

Renowned and internationally noted specialists in the field of
ultrasonics reported on the latest findings regarding the biological
interaction of ultrasound, which promised future improvements in the
methods of ultrasonic diagnostics and gave and up-to-date insight
into the biological effectiveness of ultrasound.

We are pleased to be able to publish selected contributions to
this symposium collected in one volume. The methods of investigation,
theoretical considerations and results concerning the interaction
of ultrasound on molecular, cellular and system levels contained
herein will remain up-to-date for a long time to come, providing
thought provoking material for further inter-disciplinary basic
research and medical application.

Rudolf Millner

Chairman

CONTENTS

WELCOME ADDRESS

The International Organization for Medical Physics was started to improve international communication between physical scientists throughout the world, who use their "know-how" to improve health care and medical techniques. So far, it has called six major international conferences, during which the worldwide gathering of delegates has discussed and learned of work covering the whole field of medical physics.

The Council decided recently that, in addition, it wished to sponsor smaller, more specialized symposia devoted to one carefully selected topic. This meeting is the first one to be sponsored by IOMP in accordance with this policy.

IOMP hopes that this gathering together at Reinhardsbrunn of highly qualified researchers to discuss "Ultrasound Interaction in Biology and Medicine" will prove to be of unique significance in the development of this subject, and hopes that the interchange of information will give a forward boost to your knowledge which may, in turn, help the sick wherever they are.

IOMP congratulates all those who have initiated this meeting, all those who have made the excellent preparations, and wishes it every success.

Prof. Dr. I.R. Mallard

President of the
International Organization
of Medical Physics

ULTRASONIC PROPERTIES OF BIOLOGICAL MEDIA

F. Dunn

Bioacoustics Research Laboratory
University of Illinois
Urbana, Illinois 61801, USA

INTRODUCTION

This paper comprises a brief review of the ultrasonic propagation properties of biological media, with particular attention to those properties that are considered to influence, or to be otherwise useful in, the obtaining of significant diagnostic ultrasound information and those properties important in producing and assessing biological effects. The properties are discussed according to categories which emerge readily from the reported literature[1,2]. Generalizations are then employed to characterize tissues from these categorical suggestions.

SPEED OF SOUND

Data regarding the speed of sound comes largely from measurements of freshly excised tissues[1,2]. An appreciable range appears in the reported values which is believed to result from different measuring methods being employed, from different methods of specimen preparation, and from different examples of specimens being chosen. The range of the data extends from approximately 5% for brain and muscle, to approximately 9% for fat. Nevertheless, the data show that an ordering of tissue specimens in terms of increasing speed of sound is also an ordering for increasing structural protein content, but for decreasing water content.

ATTENUATION

Because parenchymal tissues exhibit speeds of sound which are approximately the same as that for water, it has become customary to think of the soft tissues as being liquid-like media having densities and compressibilities much like water, but with significantly different attenuation and absorption behavior, viz., much greater magnitudes and a nearly linear, rather than quadratic, dependence upon frequency. However, the published literature[1,2] exhibits a very appreciable range of reported values, apparently reflecting the greater difficulty in making such measurements and in interpreting the resulting data[3,4], though it is to be noted that measurement methods and specimen preparations have improved with time and experience as publication values have decreased[5]. The reported attenuation range, in some cases, is over 100%.

ABSORPTION

There are few methods available for measuring absorption directly[4], and the transient thermoelectric method has been employed for studying freshly excised tissues as a function of frequency[6]. The exponents on frequency have been found to vary only from 1.02 to 1.08 among testis, kidney, heart, brain, liver, and tendon, even though these tissues represent substantial differences in their structural and chemical compositions. There are, however, very pronounced differences in the magnitudes of the absorption, viz., tendon being 4 to 5 times greater than liver, brain, heart, and kidney, which in turn are about twice that of testis. It should be noted that heart, brain, and kidney have approximately 16-18% protein and 1-2% collagen, and about 71-76% water. Tendon, on the other hand, has a total protein content of 35-40% with 30% collagen, but with a water content of only 63%. Testis has very little collagen, about 12% protein, but has more than 80% water. (Testis may have a greater water content than any tissue other than fetal brain.) Though brain has lesser protein content than do kidney, liver, and heart, its greater lipid and lesser collagen contents may combine in some way to provide its similar absorption properties.

The species dependence of absorption for the single organ liver from beef, pig, cat, and mouse, in the frequency range 0.5-7 MHz, all at 37°C, has been studied, and shows little, possibly negligible, difference in the observed values[6]

Comparison of these absorption measurements with the average values for attenuation taken from the literature[1,2], yields interesting contrasts[6]. Namely, there is little difference in the frequency dependence of absorption and of attenuation in the frequency range 0.5-7 MHz, suggesting that whatever the source of differences in magnitude between attenuation and absorption values (i.e., scattering, reflection, measurement artifact, etc.), that mechanism is nearly linearly dependent upon frequency. It is to be noted that the magnitudes of attenuation and absorption are greatly different, with the former being nearly a factor of three greater than the latter for each tissue.

TEMPERATURE DEPENDENCE

Measurements of the temperature dependence of attenuation of excised tissues generally yield a decreasing dependence with temperature, as is expected when dealing with a fluid viscosity mechanism. However, the situation for in vivo absorption, which is the more pertinent quantity, may be considerably different. As it is very difficult to conduct observations as a function of temperature with an ordinary mammal, because of superior temperature controlling mechanisms, measurements have been made using young mice, approximately 24 hours after birth, which are essentially poikilothermic animals[7,8]. The general demeanor of these studies is that the frequency-free absorption vs temperature comprises a family of curves whose maxima decrease and move toward ever increasing temperatures as a function of increasing frequency.

DEPENDENCE UPON CONSTITUENT MACROMOLECULES

It has long been known that the absorption of ultrasound in tissues is largely determined by the protein constituents and, because of this, aqueous solutions of globular proteins have been studied as model systems of tissue, wherein the tissue architecture may be relegated or associated with the remaining portion of the attenuation[4]. These studies have involved only globular proteins (different size/structure) which carry out the biochemical events in the physiological processes of the various organs. Studies of the ultrasonic properties of structural proteins in aqueous suspension have now been carried out[9] and it is interesting to include these results with those of globular proteins and with tissues[10]. Structural proteins provide a framework maintaining tissue structure integrity. It is to be noted that tissues comprised mainly of these proteins, mostly collagen, have much different elastic properties than do tissues having little collagen or are predominantly comprised of globular protein. Thus, it is found that values for the ultrasonic velocity of various tissues, as a function of the wet weight percentage of total protein, are contained between the two values (1) of the velocity in aqueous solutions of serum albumin (for the appropriate wet weight percentage of total protein) and (2) of the velocity in collagen suspensions. Accordingly, tissues predominantly comprised of globular protein

are expected to exhibit ultrasonic velocities near the value for
collagen-free media, with a tissue wholly so constituted exhibiting
that value for a solution of globular protein at the specified
concentration. Similarly collagenous tissues, such as tendon, where
a substantial fraction of the protein is in the form of collagen, are
expected to exhibit values well above the collagen-free, globular
protein value. This is borne out in that liver, kidney, heart, and
muscle, all with approximately the same total protein, about 17%,
of which very little, less than 1%, is collagen, have nearly the same
velocities and appear near the collagen-free value for their wet
weight percentage of total protein. Tendon, which is largely
collagen (37.6% protein, 85% of this is collagen) exhibits the
collagen value for its wet weight percentage of total protein.
Fatty tissues contain little protein and their velocities are less
than the others. Thus, it appears that the ultrasonic velocity in
tissues is governed, in some way, by the ultrasonic properties of
the individual macromolecular constituents comprising them.

Ultrasonic absorption appears to be governed by similar
relationships. That is, the absorption of tissues is found to fall
between the values, at the appropriate wet weight percentage of
total protein, of the absorption of solutions of globular proteins
and of the absorption of suspensions of collagen[10].

Thus, it appears that absorption in tissues may be considered
as a linear superposition of the absorption properties of their
protein constituents, and tissues may further appear, at least as a
first approximation, as composite materials whose ultrasonic
properties are governed by the individual ultrasonic properties of
their structural and globular protein contents.

SUMMARY

Table I is an attempt to characterize tissues according to their
ultrasonic properties and biological function at 1 MHz. Here,
tissues have been grouped, in an apparent teleologic fashion, with
a narrow range of attenuation (doubling) from group to group. It
is seen that in so doing, the velocity increases in the same direction, viz., the direction of increasing attenuation. Also,
proceeding in the same direction, tissues of ever decreasing water
content and ever increasing structural protein content become
involved. It appears, thereby, that attenuation and velocity may
characterize tissues according to functional criteria.

Possibly future detailed measurements will allow assignment of
resolvably unique values to each tissue structure, including
usefully differentiable values for pathological states, so that
attenuation and impedance values, as a function of state and of
acoustic parameters, media, etc., should specify uniquely tissues

Table 1. Average attenuation of tissues by categories

Tissue attenuation categories	Attenuation at 1 MHz (cm^{-1})	Tissue	Assumed teleology	General trends
1. Very low	0.03 0.01	serum blood	ion, metabolic, etc., transport, convection	
2. Low	0.06–0.07	adipose tissue	energy and (water) storage	
3. Medium	0.08–0.11	nervous tissue	physiological function parenchymal tissue	
	0.11 0.08–0.16 0.23 0.3	liver muscle heart kidney		
4. High	0.4	integument	structural integration, stromal tissues	
	0.5 0.6	tendon cartilage		
5. Very high	1 or more	bone (mineralized)	skeletal framework	
	>4	pulmonary tissue	gaseous exchange	

General trends:

Increasing speed of sound →

Increasing structural protein content →

← Increasing H_2O content

for diagnostic purposes. However, it is clearly not necessary to
have acoustic methods for discriminating say, between brain and
liver, but it can be seen from the figure that certain classes of
pathology should be easily identifiable and others not. For
example, cirrhosis of the liver, as manifested by collagen deposited
in place of normal tissues, could be easily identified, and is,
while metasteses of say, nerve tissue neoplasm in liver, are
probably not identifiable, at least in the early stages before
cirrhosis of the liver tissue begins. A major problem of prediction,
at present, is the paucity of available data on abnormal tissues.

REFERENCES

1. S. A. Goss, R. L. Johnston and F. Dunn, Comprehensive
      compilation of empirical ultrasonic properties of mammalian
      tissue, J. Acoust. Soc. Am. 64:423-457 (1978).
2. S. A. Goss, R. L. Johnston and F. Dunn, Compilation of empirical
      ultrasonic properties of mammalian tissues II, J. Acoust. Soc.
      Am. 68:93-108 (1980).
3. F. Dunn and W. D. O'Brien, Jr., eds., "Ultrasonic Biophysics",
      Dowden, Hutchinson & Ross, Stroudsburg (1976), Volume 7,
      Benchmark Papers in Acoustics, xix + 410 pages.
4. F. Dunn, P. D. Edmonds and W. J. Fry, Absorption and dispersion
      of ultrasound in biological media, in: "Biological Engineer-
      ing", H. P. Schwan, ed., McGraw-Hill Book Co., New York
      (1969), Chap. 3, p.205-332.
5. S. A. Goss, R. L. Johnston and F. Dunn, Ultrasound mammalian
      tissue properties literature search, Acoust. Letts. 1:171-172
      (1978).
6. S. A. Goss, L. A. Frizzell and F. Dunn, Ultrasonic absorption
      and attenuation in mammalian tissues, Ultrasound Med. Biol.
      5:181-186 (1979).
7. F. Dunn and J. K. Brady, Pogloshchenie ul'trazvyeks v
      biologicheskikh sredakh (Ultrasonic absorption in biological
      media), Biofizika 18:1063-1066 (1973), in Russian, English
      abstract. English translation: Biophysics 18:1128-1132 (1974).
8. F. Dunn and J. K. Brady, Temperature and frequency dependence
      of ultrasonic absorption in tissue, in: "Proceedings of the
      8th International Congress on Acoustics", Goldcrest Press,
      Trowbridge, Wilts. (1974), Volume 1, 366c.
9. S. A. Goss and F. Dunn, Ultrasonic propagation properties of
      collagen, Phys. Med. Biol. 25:827-837 (1980).
10. S. A. Goss, L. A. Frizzell, F. Dunn and K. A. Dines, Dependence
      of the ultrasonic properties of biological tissue on
      constituent proteins, J. Acoust. Soc. Am. 67:1041-1044 (1980).

TRANSDUCERS AND SOUNDFIELDS

L. Filipczynski

Institute of Fundamental Technological Research
Polish Academy of Science
00-049 Warsaw, Poland

The purpose of this paper is to present and to discuss some fundamental problems and solutions connected with piezoelectric transducers and soundfields generated for ultrasonic medical applications.

The first problem I should like to review is the generation of soundfields with piezoelectric transducers. To obtain sufficient bandwidth, power and sensitivity the transducer must be carefully designed to be properly coupled with the electronic transmitter and receiver and with the biological medium in which ultrasonic waves propagate.

The theory of ultrasonic transducers performing thickness expander vibrations was given by Mason and is based on a one-dimensional approach[1]. As a consequence many authors apply Mason's electromechanical equivalent circuit but others have shown experimentally that the vibration patterns are very complex and do not resemble one-dimensional vibrations[2]. Fig. 1.(A) shows displacement (amplitude and phase) distributions measured on the transducer's surface along its diameter[3]. The transducer vibrated freely in thickness resonances near to 1.6 MHz. This is not possible to explain using Mason's circuit.

However, we could show[3] -- using the capacitance measurement method -- that with the increase of the mechanical load on the transducer's back surface the many resonances amalgamate to one resonance and the transducer's surface vibrates like a piston (Fig. 1.(B) and (C)). Hence in diagnostical applications -- where the transducer's back surface must be heavily loaded for obtaining a short pulse -- the one-dimensional approach and Mason's circuit are fully justified.

7

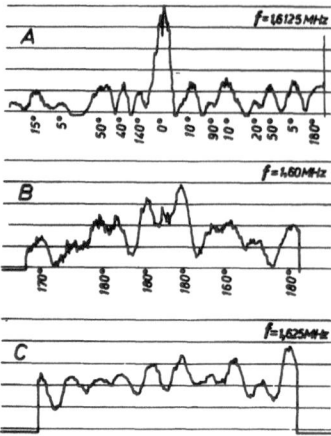

Fig. 1. Displacement distribution measured along the diameter of a
         ceramic transducer, vibrating freely (A), loaded on its
         back surface with perspex (B), and with tungsten-plastic
         composition (C). In the last case phase differences were
         lower than 5°.

         Fig. 2.(A) presents Mason's circuit which can be easily trans-
formed to the form (Fig. 2.(B)) which is very useful for transient
analysis[4]. One can see that in the case of electrical pulse
excitation (at the terminals situated in the lower part of Fig. 2.)
one obtains at the same time two mechanical pulses on the resistors
R_A and R_B which correspond to media loading the transducer on its

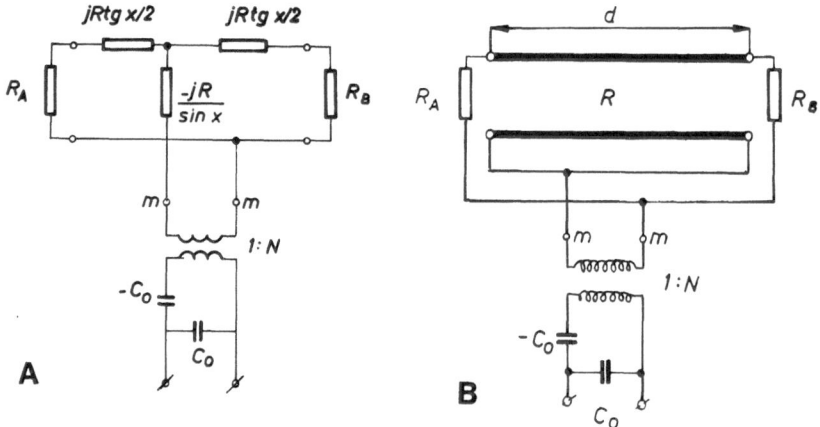

Fig. 2. A -- Mason's equivalent circuit for piezoelectric
              transducer
         B -- the same for transient analysis

back and front surfaces. This could be shown[5] in the experiment
presented in Fig. 3. This phenomenon can be easily explained in
Fig. 4. The uniform electric field when applied to the transducer
has the effect that in all its segments there arise mechanical
stresses, which try to expand every segment and to displace its
boundaries. However, on every boundary two stresses are acting from
opposite sides. As they are equal and opposite in direction they
cancel themselves out. Only on both transducers' surfaces there is
no counter-balance of stresses and displacements must arise. In this
way one can describe transients in the transducer, however, only
under the limiting condition that the electrical terminals are
open[4]. So we are able to understand the mechanism of transients

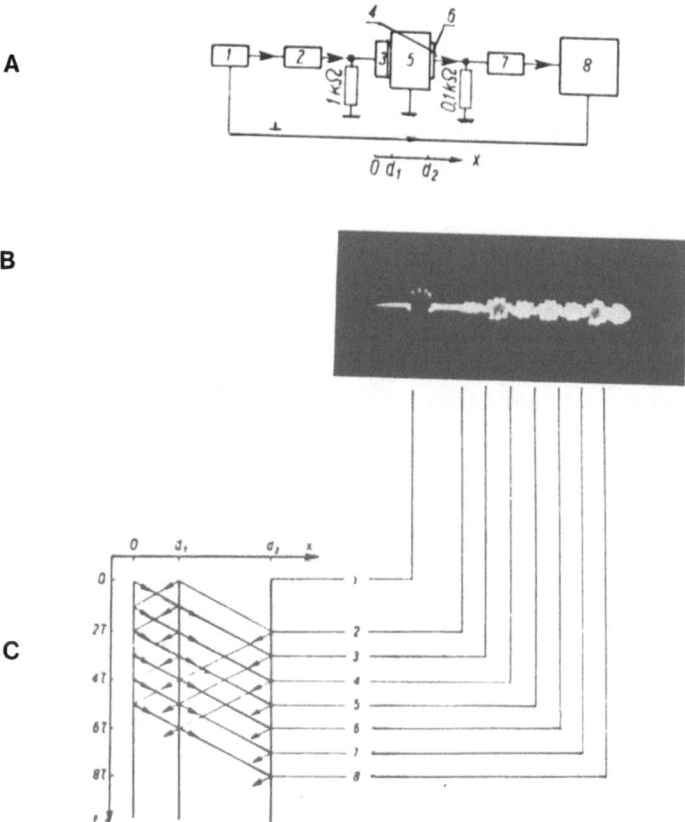

A

B

C

Fig. 3. A -- Experiment with a thick quartz[6] excited with a short
             h.f. pulse and transmitting many ultrasonic pulses
             through the sample[4] to the thin receiving quartz[7].
         B -- Electrical pulse and ultrasonic pulses radiated by
             both quartz surfaces.
         C -- x,t diagram explaining the origin of the observed
             pulses.

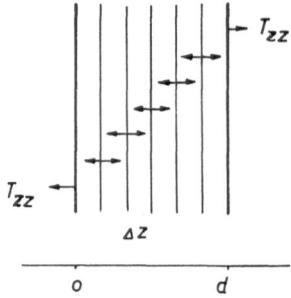

Fig. 4. Stresses T_{zz} in the piezoelectric transducer
d - Trandsucer's thickness

and the function of special transducers with nonuniform electrical
fields. Mason's circuit makes it possible to compute the exact
form of ultrasonic pulses radiated into the biological medium
assuming various types of mechanical and electrical loadings,
matching layers and so on.

Using the Laplace transform, four terminal network theory and
the FFT transform one can compute many practical cases as shown for
the electrical excitation in the form of the Heaviside step function
of 250 V amplitude[8]. Fig. 5. presents the pulse transmitted into
the soft tissue and then received by the same transducer with a
medium load on its back surface. One obtains 5 V electrical input
on the electronic receiver. A biological medium with no attenuation
and no diffraction losses were assumed in this case. For the same
transducer with a $\lambda/4$ matching layer the pulse is shorter and its
amplitude is 4 times higher. Fig. 6. presents the pulse for the
transducer ideally matched on its back surface. Interesting is the
wedge transducer given by Alfonso[9], for which one obtains a short
pulse even with no back loading. There is also another way of
shortening the pulse length possible by changing the electrical
excitation pulse shape[10].

I have briefly described the generation of ultrasonic pulses
of a short duration time which makes it possible to obtain the
axial resolution high enough for diagnostic systems. For special
purposes like ultrasonic spectroscopy it is necessary and possible
to generate much shorter pulses using also piezoelectric materials
with high internal absorption like lead niobate.

The next fundamental problem of ultrasonic diagnostic systems
is the lateral resolution which depends on soundfield formation.
The first improvement in this field was to focus acoustically the
ultrasonic beam using plane transducers with a plastic lens or
concave transducers. The simplest method to compute this kind of
ultrasonic field was to use the well known Rayleigh formula[11]

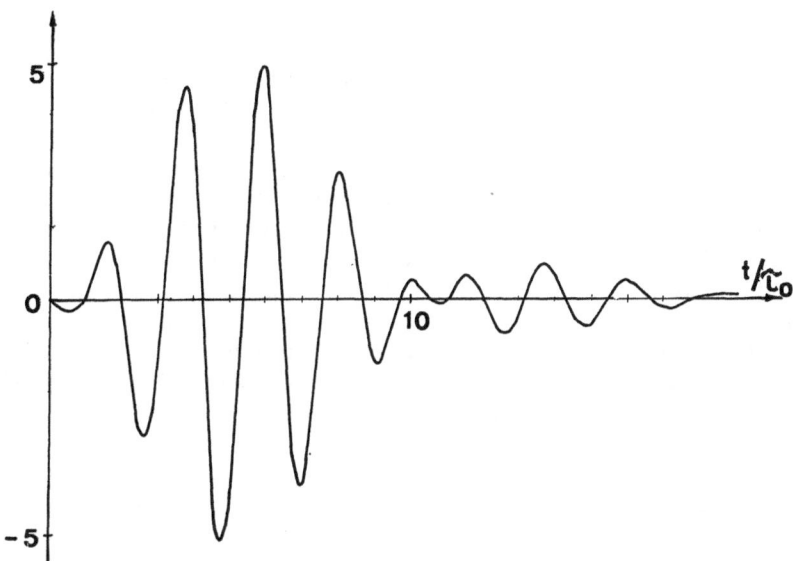

Fig. 5.   Pulse shape in the case of the transducer with a medium
load on its back surface.

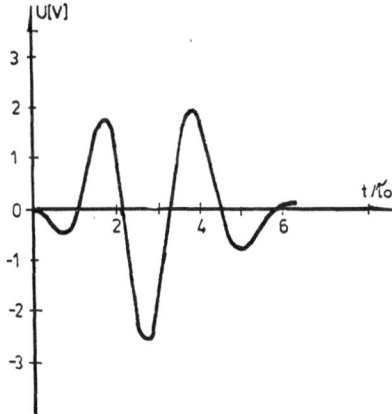

Fig. 6.   The same case as in Fig. 5.; however, the transducer's
back surface ideally matched.

which may be considered a quantitative formulation of the Huygens' principle

$$p = \frac{j\omega\rho}{2\pi} \int_S v(\frac{e^{-jkt}}{t}) \, dS \qquad\qquad k = \omega/c$$

where p denotes acoustical pressure, S vibrating surface, v its velocity, r distance. It is valid exactly only for plane vibrating surfaces. However, it may be used also for weak focussing transducers neglecting the elementary waves first radiated and then reflected at the edges of the radiating transducer. However, experimental and theoretical field distributions show a rather good agreement in this case (Fig. 7.) Interesting properties are shown by beams radiated with plane or weak focussing transducers having Gaussian velocity distributions on their surfaces[7]. The maxima and minima of amplitude and phase which are present when the velocity distribution is uniform do not appear in the ultrasonic beam (Fig. 8.) There are also no side lobes existing.

However, a dramatic increase in the lateral resolution of diagnostic devices is possible with a dynamic and aperture controlling systems by means of advanced electronic and transducer technology and design. Fig. 9. presents our disc transducer composed of many

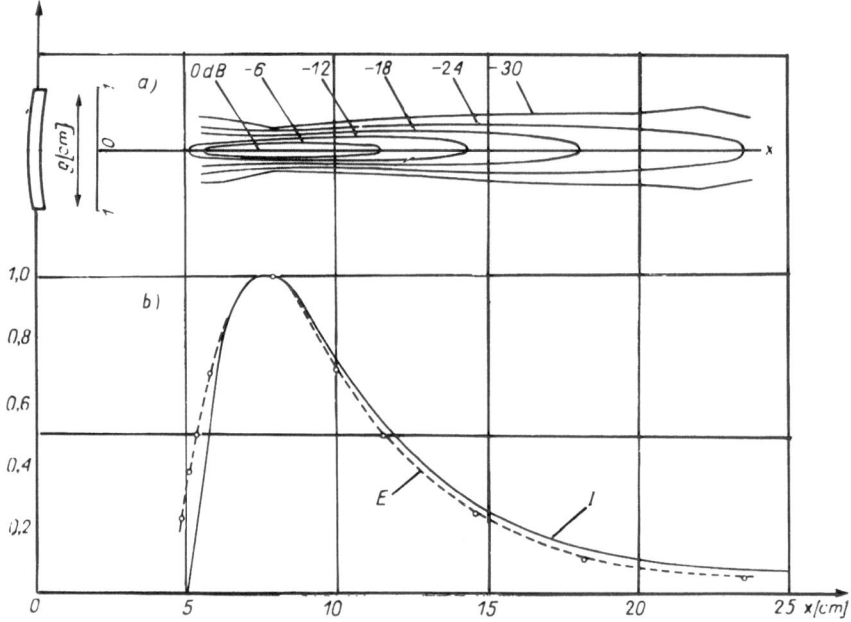

Fig. 7.   Intensity distribution in the ultrasonic field of weak
          focussing transducer.
          I - calculated, E - measured

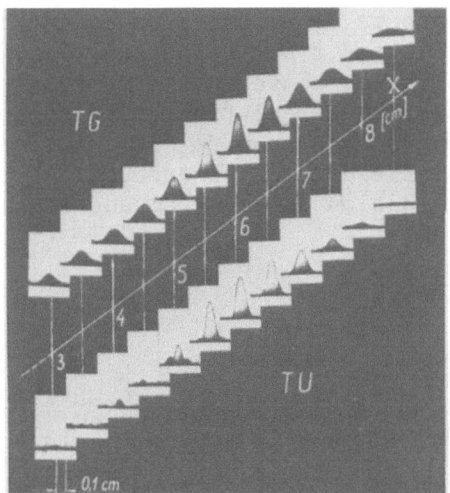

Fig. 8. Measurement results of ultrasonic fields radiated by weak focussing transducers with Gaussian (TG) and uniform (TU) velocity distributions on their surfaces.

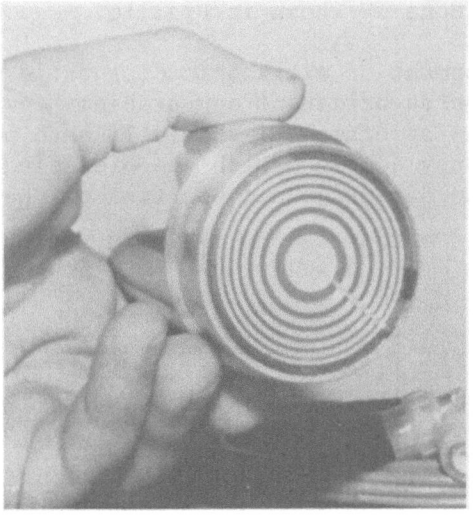

Fig. 9. Disc transducer composed of 7 radiating elements.

rings excited electronically with variable time delays which make
it possible to form and to shift the focus along the beam axis with
the wave velocity.

In this way the focus is always situated at the point where it
is expected to be reflected from the pulse. Fig. 10 shows the
beamwidth obtained with the above system for a distance of 24 cm
divided into 5 zones. The calculations were performed for steady
state, however, they can also be made for transients. The acoustic
potential in the soundfield can be presented[12] as the convolution
of the velocity distribution on the transducer and the delta response
function of the system

$$\phi(\vec{r},t) = v(t)*h(7,t)$$

where the delta response function is

$$h(\vec{r},t) = \begin{cases} c & \text{for } \frac{z}{c} < t < \frac{R'}{c} \\ \frac{c}{\pi} \arccos \left[\frac{c^2t^2+r_o^2-Q^2z^2}{2r_o\sqrt{c^2t^2-z^2}} \right] & \frac{R'}{c} < t < \frac{R}{c} \\ o & t < \frac{z}{c} \text{ and } t > \frac{R}{c} \end{cases}$$

z denotes the distance on the transducer's axis, R/R' the max/min
distance, r_o the distance from the transducer's axis, c the wave
velocity. From the above formulae we are able to compute the
spatial distribution of the soundfield of the system from Fig. 9.
when radiating short pulses (Fig. 11.). The presented result
corresponds to the zone IV shown in Fig. 10.

A rapid development of ultrasonic diagnostic methods and
instrumentation creates permanent new problems for both transducers
and soundfields. As an example I should like to present in Fig. 12.
the idea of the biopsy needle N with the piezoelectric transducer T
controlling both the direction and position of the needle by means

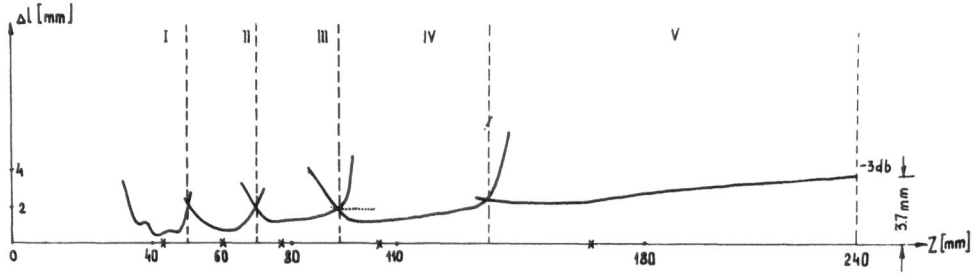

Fig. 10. Beamwidth (mm) of the transducer shown in Fig. 9. as the
          function of the distance Z from the transducer (wavelength
          0.63 mm).

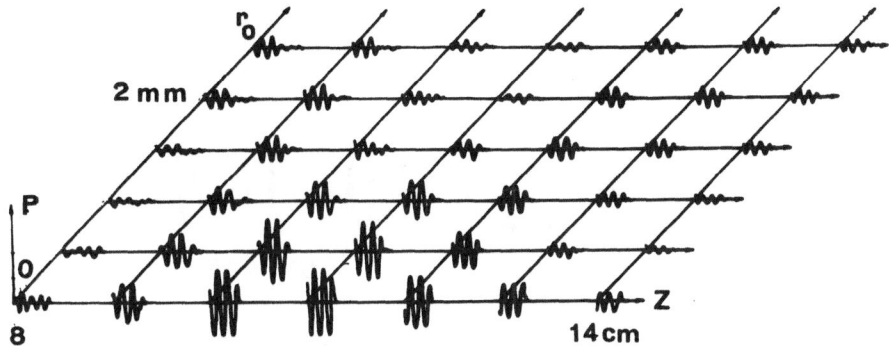

Fig. 11. Spatial distribution of the soundfield radiated by the
          system of Fig. 9. for short pulses.
          Z - the distance on the tranducer's axis
          r_0 - the distance perpendicular to the transducer's axis

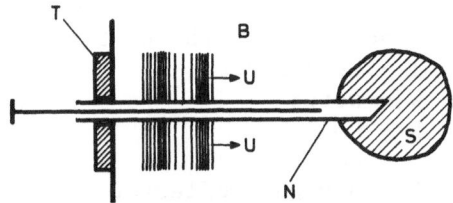

Fig. 12. Idea of the biopsy needle.
          S - structure under examination

of ultrasonic waves U while inserting it into the patient's body B.
Fig. 13. presents experiments with the needle performed in water[6].
On the bottom left-hand side, one can see the arrangement with a
perspex reflector P which gives a high echo on the echoscope screen.
One can observe also the echo from the end of the needle. When the
needle is shifted to the left in the X direction the end echo changes
its position in the same direction. However, it is interesting to
observe -- on the right-hand side -- the same phenomenon when
shifting the rod R to the left, which is inserted into the needle.
This is the evidence that the wave propagating along the needle
penetrates into the needle interior. We could not find any other
wave propagating, for instance with the velocity as for metal. One
could show that in this case a kind of surface wave propagates with
a velocity which is only slightly lower than that in water.

The problem is far from being solved definitively, however, it
shows how unexpectedly new problems arise in the soundfield domain
when developing ultrasonic diagnostic methods.

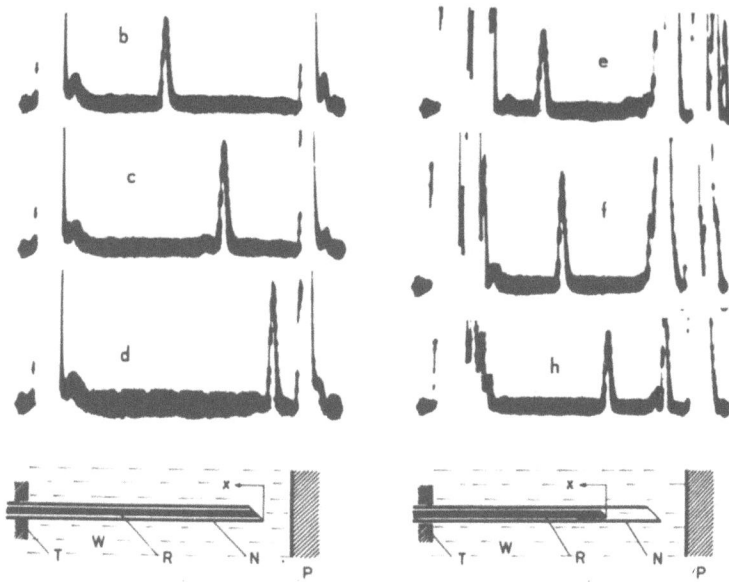

Fig. 13.   Experiments with the biopsy needle.
          T - transducer
          W - water
          R - rod
          N - needle
          P - perspex reflector

REFERENCES

1. W. P. Mason, "Electromechanical Transducers and Wave Filters",
    Van Nostrand, Princeton (1948).
2. E. A. G. Shaw, Vibration patterns of loaded barium titanate and
    quartz discs, J. Acoust. Soc. Am. 32:1463 (1960).
3. G. Lypacewicz and L. Filipczynski, Measurement method and
    experimental study of ceramic transducer vibrations, Acustica
    24:216 (1971).
4. L. Filipczynski, Transients, equivalent circuit and negative
    capacitance of a piezoelectric transducer performing thickness
    vibrations, J. Tech. Phys. 16:121 (1975).
5. L. Filipczynski, Properties of the X cut quartz tranducer loaded
    with a solid medium, in: "Proc. II Conf. Ultrasonics", Polish
    Academy of Sciences, Warsaw (1957), p.35.
6. L. Filipczynski, Ultrasonic wave propagation along the surface
    of a rod in water, Archives of Acoustics 4:271 (1979).
7. L. Filipczynski and J. Etienne, Theoretical study and experiments
    on spherical focussing transducers with Gaussian surface
    velocity distribution, Acustica 28:121 (1973).

8. A. Markiewicz, Analysis of tranceiving pulse systems used in
    medical diagnostics, Archiwum Akustyki 15:207 (1980).
9. G. Alphons , The wedged transducer, in: "Ultrasound in Medicine,
    Vol. 3B: Engineering Aspects", D. White and R. Brown, eds.,
    Plenum, New York (1977).
10. V. Domarkas and R. Kazys, "Piezoelectric Transducers for Measuring
    Devices", Mintis, Vilnius (1975), in Russian.
11. Lord Rayleigh, "Theory of Sound", London (1926).
12. P. R. Stephanishen, Transient radiation from pistons in an
    infinite planar baffle, J. Acoust. Soc. Am. 49:1629 (1971).
13. M. Hubelbank and O. Tretiak, Focussed ultrasonic transducer
    design, MIT Res. Lab. Elec. Q.P.R. 98:169 (1971).

MEASUREMENT OF ULTRASONIC POWER WITH THE RADIATION FORCE AND

THERMOBALANCE METHOD*

F. Holzer and P. Wach

Institute of Biomedical Engineering
Technical University of Graz
A-8010 Graz, Inffeldgasse 18, Austria

INTRODUCTION

There is a growing number of studies published in the literature which are devoted to the problem of the possible hazards in the medical applications of ultrasound. It is important to note that sufficient and conclusive evidence, on which the safety of medical ultrasound may be reasonably questioned, can only be obtained, if the ultrasonic field used in the experiment is properly defined and the relevant parameters are measured. In this connection, the measurement of the average acoustic power emitted by an ultrasonic transducer and the improvement of the related measuring methods are of fundamental importance.

In the following, first we will present a very short theoretical approach to the radiation force method, based on the HAMILTON-JACOBI theory of continuous systems. Then, we will briefly outline the theoretical foundations of the thermobalance method and give some experimental results.

RADIATION FORCE METHOD

Let us consider the situation which is schematically illustrated in Fig. 1. An ultrasonic beam emitted from a transducer propagates adiabatically in an ideal liquid and is completely

*This work is supported by the Austrian Foundation for the Support of Scientific Research, project no. 4089

19

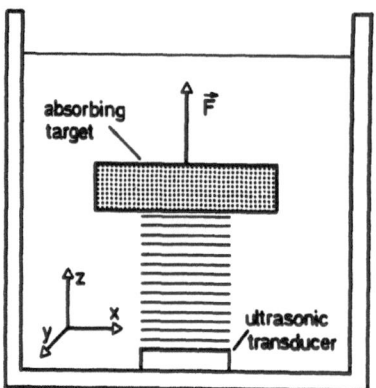

Fig. 1. Ultrasonic irradiation of an absorbing target immersed in
a liquid.

intercepted and absorbed by a target. Consequently, there is a
transport of acoustic energy and of acoustic momentum into the
absorbing target, where the energy is converted into heat and the
momentum is converted into force.

Now, let the densities of energy and momentum of the beam be
defined by E and M, respectively.

Then, from the HAMILTON-JACOBI theory[1,2] we can obtain the
result that the phase velocity, c, is defined by

$$c = \frac{E}{M} \; .$$ (1)

The momentum flux density, i.e., the amount of momentum
streaming in unit time through the unit area of the target's surface,
is defined by

$$T = Mc = E \; ,$$ (2)

whereby equation (1) is used.

In the same way we obtain the energy flux density, or intensity,
namely

$$I = Ec = \frac{P}{A} \; ,$$ (3)

where P is the power and A is the cross-sectional area of the beam.
Now, since the beam is completely absorbed, the time-rate of
momentum transport into the target, TA, is equal to the time-rate
of momentum change. From Newton's second law then it follows that

force

$$F = TA = \frac{P}{c} \tag{4}$$

is exerted on the target. All magnitudes in this derivation are, obviously, averaged in space and time.

It should be stressed that equation (1) holds for every type of radiation* and that the final result in equation (4) is valid also for dispersive media.

THERMOBALANCE METHOD

In addition to the phenomenon of radiation force, the buoyancy of the target is increased by thermal expansion, which is caused by the conversion of acoustic energy into heat.

Fig. 2. schematically shows the transport of energy occurring in the region of the target. Let Q_1 and Q_2 be the amount of energy entering and leaving the target, respectively. Then we can write

$$dQ_1 = Pdt \text{ and } dQ_2 = a\Delta Tdt \ , \tag{5}, (6)$$

where P is the absorbed ultrasonic power, $\Delta T = T_1 - T_2$ the difference of the temperatures inside and outside the target, and a is a constant factor. Then the energy

$$dQ = dQ_1 - dQ_2 = mCdt \tag{7}$$

remains inside the target, where m is the mass and C is the specific heat of the target. Combining equations (5), (6) and (7), we have

$$dT = \frac{1}{mC} (P - a\Delta T) \ dt \ . \tag{8}$$

Assuming that T_2 remains constant, integration of equation (8) yields

$$-\frac{1}{a} \ln(P - a\Delta T) = \frac{1}{mC} t + const \ . \tag{9}$$

If ΔT is assumed to be zero for t=0, we obtain

$$\Delta T_{(t)} = \frac{P}{a} (1 - e^{-\frac{a}{mC} t}) \ . \tag{10}$$

If the buoyancy of the target is assumed to depend linearly on its

---

*If a stream of particles is considered, c of course is not the velocity of phase, but the velocity of propagation of surfaces of constant action[1].

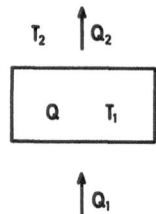

Fig. 2. Transport of energy occurring in the region of the
         absorbing target.

temperature, namely

$$\Delta F (t) = b\Delta T (t) ,$$

we can write

$$\Delta F = \alpha (1-e^{-\beta t}) \tag{11}$$

with the abbreviations

$$\alpha = \frac{b}{a}p \text{ and } \beta = \frac{a}{mc} . \tag{12}$$

Fig. 3. shows a typical pen-recorder chart of the apparent
weight of an absorbing target which is immersed in water and
suspended from one arm of a microbalance (weight decreases from
bottom to top). At point "ON", the ultrasound, which is upwardly

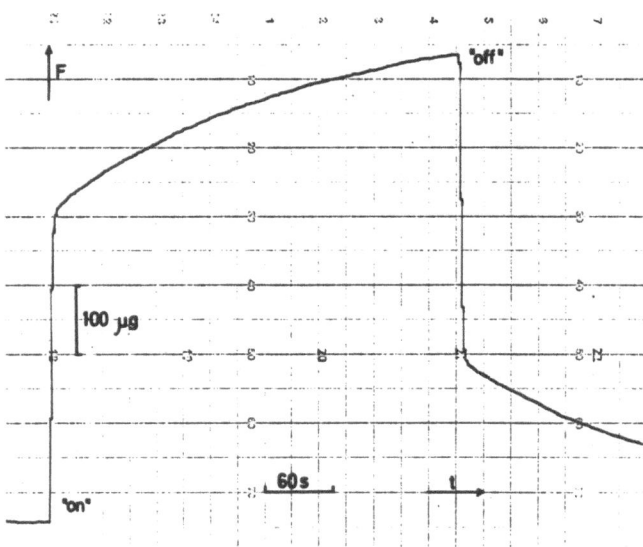

Fig. 3. Apparent weight of an absorbing target immersed in water,
         weight decreases from bottom to top.

emitted from a transducer located below the target, is switched on.
The rapid rise of the readout is caused by the radiation force
exerted on the target, while the slow is a consequence of the thermal
expansion of the target.

Similarly, at point "OFF", the ultrasound is switched off, the
radiation force rapidly disappears and the target "cools down".
The steps in the recorder line are due to strobed digital-to-analog
conversion.

Now, the same experiment illustrated in Fig. 3. allows the
determination of the ultrasonic power by two independent methods.
The first is the well known radiation force method. In this case,
the radiation force value is graphically determined from the chart
and then introduced, in appropriate units, into equation (4).

The second method is what we call the thermobalance method.
Here, the experimental values of the change of buoyancy, i.e., the
apparent weight of the target between the points "ON" and "OFF",
minus the radiation force and the extrapolated zero-line-values,
are introduced into equation (11) and the factors   and   are
calculated by the least square method.

Since from equation (12) we obtain the expression

$$P = \alpha\beta L ,$$
(13)

the ultrasonic power of the beam can be determined by introducing
α and β into equation (13), if the calibration factor L is known.

For a homogeneous material we find

$$L = \frac{mc}{b} = \frac{\rho_M \cdot c}{\rho_L \gamma g} ,$$
(14)

where ρ_M and γ are the density and the coefficient of thermal
expansion of the material of the target, respectively. ρ_L is the
density of the surrounding liquid and g is the constant of gravity.

Fig. 4. shows an example of application of the thermobalance
method. The crosses represent the experimental values, while the
line is the theoretical function with the figures of α and β as
indicated. The power level in this example is about 7 mW.

Due to the excellent agreement between experiment and theory
we can conclude that the physical model of Fig. 2., used for the
theoretical derivation, represents a sufficient approximation of
the real process.

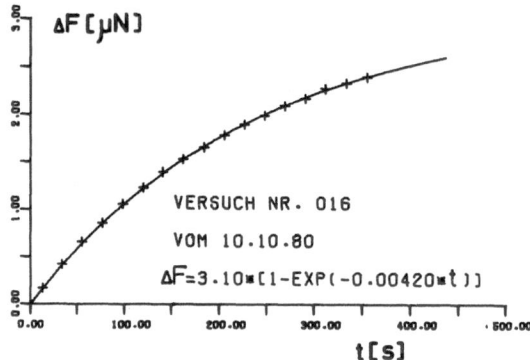

Fig. 4.   Application of the thermobalance method. Experimental
          values of the change of buoyancy have been fitted to the
          theoretical curve defined by equation (12) by the least
          square method.

RESULTS

     The measuring system, which is schematically illustrated in
Fig. 5., is quite similar to other apparatus described in the
literature[3,4]

     Relative power measurements were performed using a rubber target,
absolute results were obtained by a castor oil target with a
calibration constant of 291400 $\frac{Ws}{N}$, at an estimated error of about
20%. The thermobalance results were typically about 15% above the
corresponding radiation force result, and, hence, within the limits
of the stated calibration error.

     The reproducibility of the thermobalance results is character-
ized by a standard deviation of 3% for 10 consecutive measurements
at a power level of 7 mW.

     Work is in progress at our institute in order to reduce the
systematic error of the calibration constant and to improve the
stability of the driving circuit and, hence, the reproducibility of
the method. With the present experimental system we found no
significant difference between nearfield and farfield measurements
or between flat or focussed transducers.

     In conclusion, we can say that the thermobalance method allows
independent and absolute measurements of ultrasonic power in the
mW-range. According to the principle of the method, which is the
conversion of acoustic energy into heat, it is independent of the
shape and direction of incidence of the ultrasonic beam. This is
the main advantage of this method compared to the radiation force
method. On the other hand, excellent thermal and electrical stability for about 5 minutes is required, which at the moment limits the
reproducibility of the method.

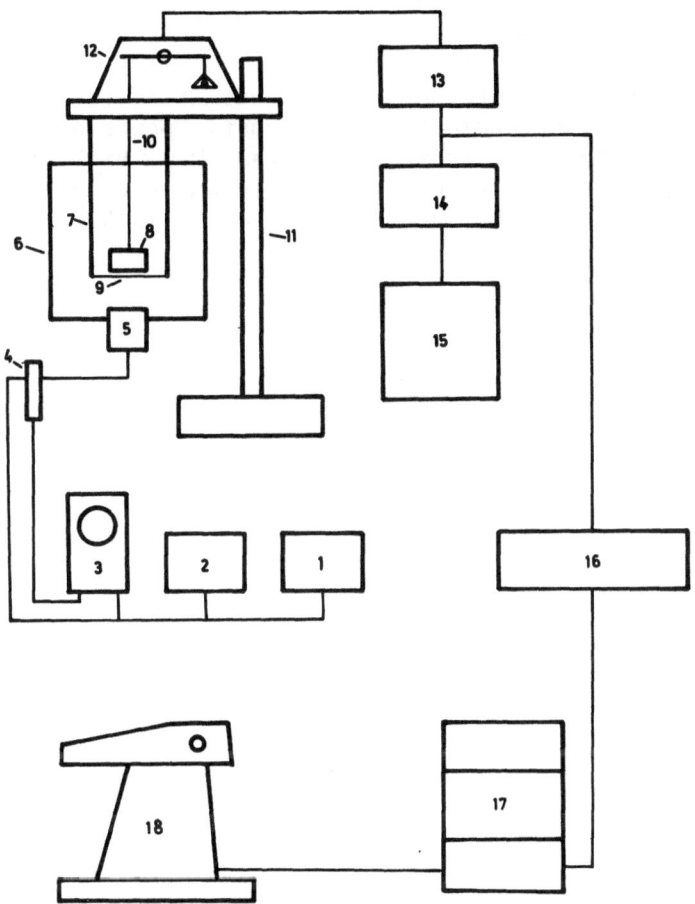

Fig. 5. Experimental set-up used for measuring ultrasonic power by
         the radiation force and the thermobalance method.

1.	function generator	10.	hanging wire
2.	frequency counter	11.	balance support
3.	oscilloscope	12.	microbalance
4.	snap-on ammeter	13.	balance control unit
5.	transducer	14.	d/a converter
6.	outer vessel	15.	x-t pen-recorder
7.	inner vessel	16.	computer interface
8.	absorbing target	17.	computer
9.	shielding membrane	18.	teletype

REFERENCES

1. H. Rund, "The Hamilton-Jacobi Theory and the Calculus of
    Variations", Van Nostrand, London (1966).
2. P. Wach, F. Holzer, N. Leitgeb and S. Schuy, On the theory of
    acoustic radiation force and its application in ultrasonic
    power measurements, manuscript submitted to Acustica.
3. J. A. Rooney, Determination of acoustic power outputs in the
    microwatt-milliwatt range, Ultras. Med. Biol. 1:241 (1973).
4. K. Brendel, Probleme der Messung kleiner Ultraschalleistungen,
    in: "DAGA 75", VDI Verlag Düsseldorf (1975), p.581.

TRANSMITTER CHARACTERISTICS OF ULTRASOUND BROAD-BAND TRANSDUCERS FOR ULTRASONIC SPECTROSCOPY

N. Leitgeb

Institute of Biomedical Engineering
Technical University of Graz
A-8010 Graz, Inffeldgasse 18, Austria

and K.-P. Richter

Institute of Applied Biophysics
Martin-Luther-University Halle
DDR-4014 Halle, Strasse der DSF 81, GDR

INTRODUCTION

Ultrasonic transducers play a major role in ultrasonic diagnosis. Their transfer characteristics and emitted ultrasonic field determine to a considerable degree the quality of A-scans as well as B-scan pictures. For the application of methods of tissue differentiation such as signal processing techniques and ultrasonic spectroscopy, special broad-band transducers with high sensitivity and a known ultrasonic field were developed and their transmitter characteristics were measured.

DESIGN AND ELECTRO-MECHANIC PROPERTIES

A circular piezoceramic disc is used as the active element of the transducers. Generally, ceramic transducers are matched with tissue impedance and directly damped at the back of the ceramic disc. Sensitivity as well as bandwidth can be improved by multiple matching layers. However, for technological reasons two layers have proved to have special advantages. To calculate theoretically the impulse response function or the transfer function, the transducer system was treated as an acoustic transmission line. Acoustic impedances and layer thickness could then be calculated

and ultrasonic transducers with center frequencies between 1 and 8 MHz
and two λ/4-matching layers could be constructed[1]. The bandwidths
amount to 60-70% of the center frequency. As a measure of the
acoustic properties the frequency dependence of the electrical
admittance was used, as it could be checked easily by experiment after
it had been theoretically calculated.

MEASUREMENTS

To study the transmitting properties of the transducers, an
extensive measurement program was carried through. The results are
compared with those of commercial transducers. The measurements
comprised:

(a) measurement of the transmitter characteristics in pulsed mode,
     by computer-controlled scanning along a half sphere with a
     stepping motor driven measurement arrangement,

(b) measurement of the axial and lateral sound pressure distribution,
     by scanning with micromanipulators,

(c) measurement of the sound beam geometry in a plane through the
     beam axis, by computer-controlled scanning in cartesian
     coordinates with a stepping motor driven measurement arrangement,

(d) measurement of the temporal and spatial averaged sonic power
     as a function of frequency, by the radiation force method.

The relative measurement of the sound pressure was performed using
a hydrophone (Medisonic), the ceramic diameter of which was 0.5 mm.
To avoid standing waves, the hydrophone was surrounded with an
absorbing target. All measurements were performed in degassed water,
the temperature of which was constant at 19°C.

The analysis of the received ultrasonic rf signals was performed
with a computer. For digitization a transient-recorder with a
sample frequency of 20 MHz was used. According to its 4 K 8-bit-
buffer memory 204.8 μs time signals could be recorded. The measured
transducers were excited either by 580 V voltage peaks from an ultrasonic diagnostic device (Kretz) or for cw-measurements by a frequency
generator.

To measure the spatial transmitter characteristics, the sound
field was scanned along a half sphere around the transmitter by a
hydrophone, which was moved along vertical and horizontal circles
by computer-controlled stepping motors[2]. To improve accuracy the
power spectra of the received signals were used to compute the
average signal power, which was used as the parameter, rather than
the peak echo amplitude. The measurement result for a broad-band

transducer is compared in Fig. 1. with a commercial 2 MHz-transducer.
Even if one takes into account that for the 2 MHz-transducer the
signal peak amplitudes are plotted, one can see that the broad-band
transducer exhibits a considerably improved side lobe suppression.

The measurement of the spatial transmitter characteristic
provides a comprehensive survey of the transmitting properties of
the transducers and shows the degree of the rotational symmetry of
the transmitted sound field.

The dependence of the sound pressure in different ranges
however, was studied by measuring the lateral profiles with a smaller
spatial sample interval. For the measurements micromanipulators
were used.

Fig. 2. shows the sound pressure profiles for a commercial small
band transducer (Kretz) with a nominal center frequency of 4 MHz
cw sinus signals. Although the measurements show good results in the
far field range, in spite of the small dimensions of the hydrophone in

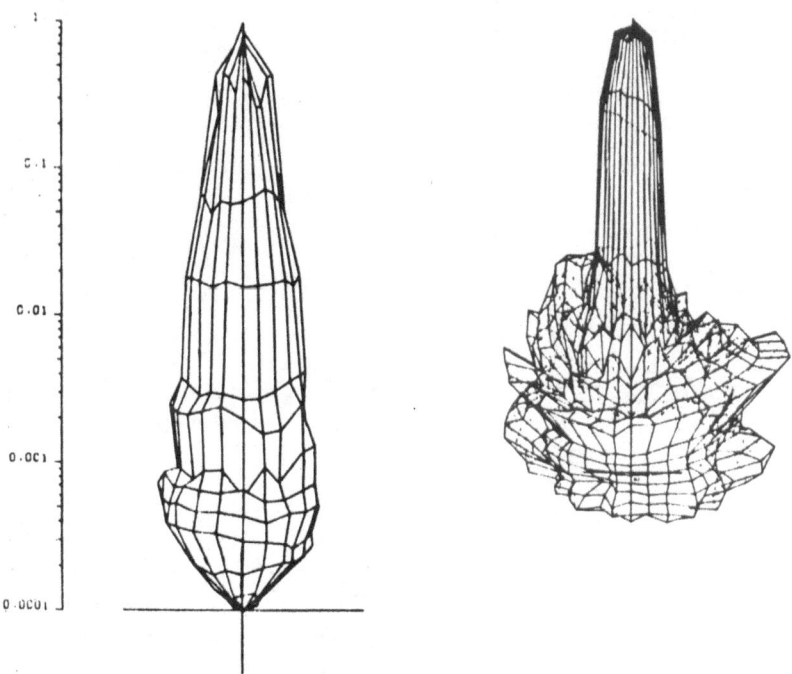

Fig. 1.   Spatial distribution of the mean signal power for a broad-
           band transducer (left) and spatial distribution of the
           signal peak amplitude for a commercial 2 MHz-transducer,
           in a logarithmic scale.

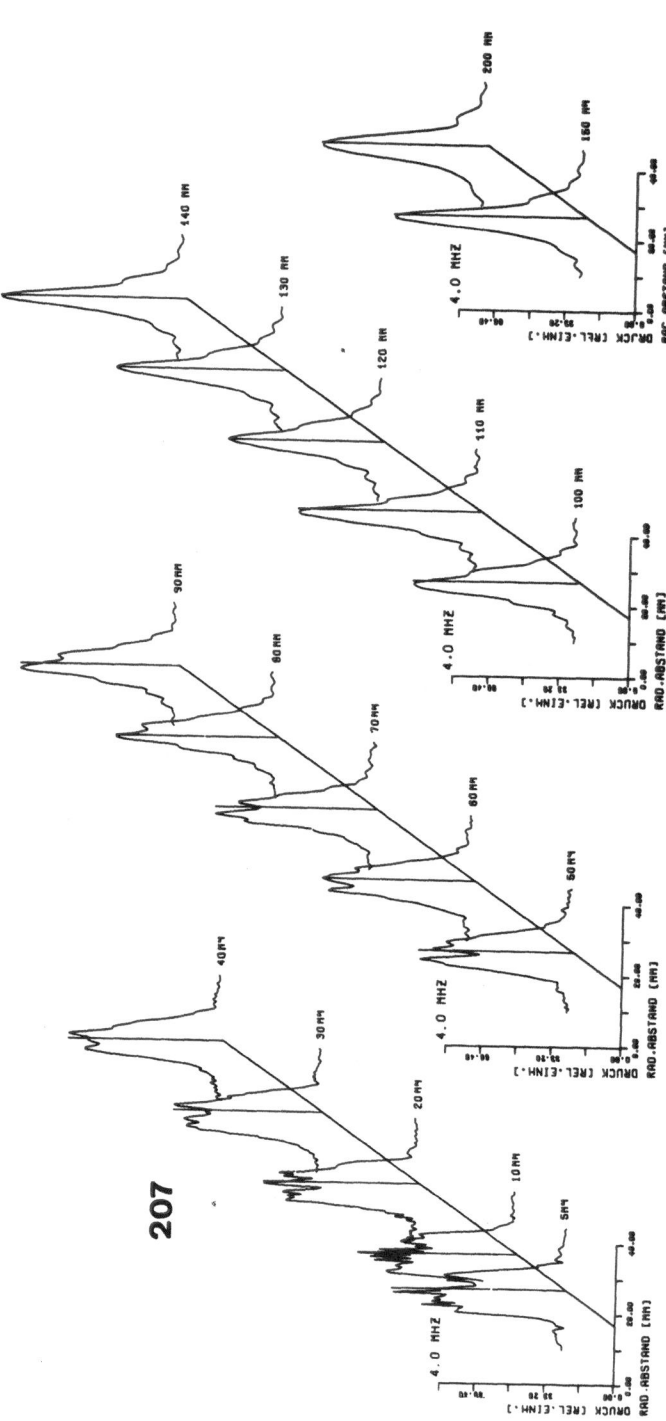

Fig. 2. Lateral sound pressure profiles of a 4 MHz center frequency small band transducer, with a
4 MHz cw-excitation.

the near field, with rapid changing pressure maxima and minima the
measured signals are low pass filtered due to the integration over
the transducer crystal.

To study the spectral composition of the transmitter signals
dependent on range, the transmitter was impulse excited. The
received signals were digitized and their spectra computed by FFT
analysis. The lateral distribution of these power spectra is shown
in Fig. 3. for measurements in 40, 80 and 120 mm distance, from the
broad-band transducer. For increased visibility the mean power of
only 10 frequency bands is plotted.

It could be shown by these measurements that due to different
transmission behavior for the various frequency components, and
perhaps due to nonlinear effects of sound propagation, the spectral
composition of the transmitted signals is not constant even within
the main lobe. With increased lateral distance this effect increases
considerably.

Especially for quantitative analysis of ultrasonic signals in
medical diagnostics, the determination of the range dependent sound
lobes is important to estimate the dimensions of the sample volumes.
For this purpose the sound pressure distribution along a plane
through the sound beam axis was measured at cw-excitation, by scanning in cartesian coordinates with a computer-controlled scanning
arrangement. To decrease time sampling errors the mean values of
102.4 µs-windowed sinus signals were computed. Spatial sampling
intervals were 1.5 mm lateral and 6 mm axial, starting at a range
of 10 mm from the transducer. For analysis of an area of 90 x 140 mm
therefore 1464 single measurements at each investigated frequency
were necessary.

Fig. 4. shows the results for the broad-band transducer for the
frequency range 1-8 MHz. In Figs. 5. and 6. the distributions for
commercial transducers with nominal center frequencies of 4 MHz and
2 MHz respectively are presented.

The comparison with the broad-band transducer not only shows
a broader beam width and therefore a worse lateral resolution but
a lower side band suppression of the small band transducers, which
was indicated by the spatial transducer measurements in Fig. 1.
too.

The different width of the ultrasonic main lobes is demonstrated
in Fig. 7. by a quantitative comparison where points of equal pressure decrease relative to the main lobe maximum dependent on range
were connected.

The dependence of the 3 dB-width of the main lobe on the
excitation frequency is shown in Fig. 8., for the broad-band
transducer.

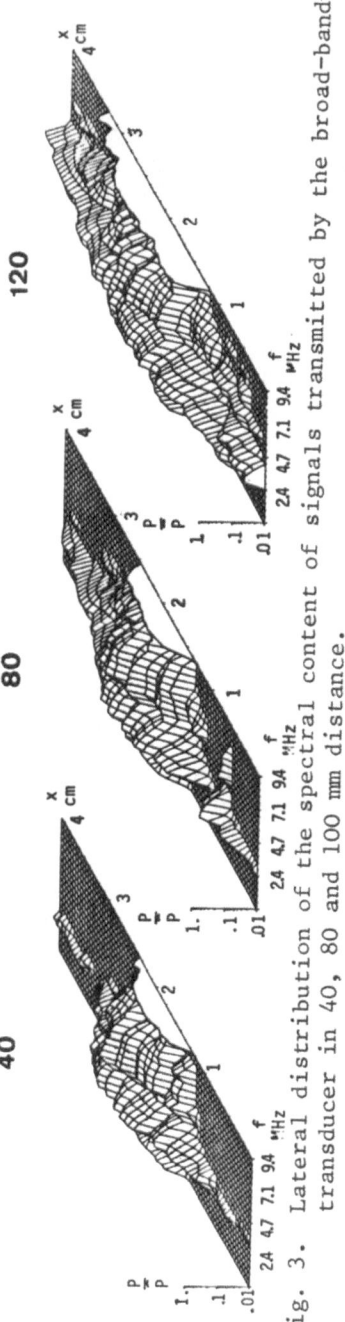

Fig. 3. Lateral distribution of the spectral content of signals transmitted by the broad-band transducer in 40, 80 and 100 mm distance.

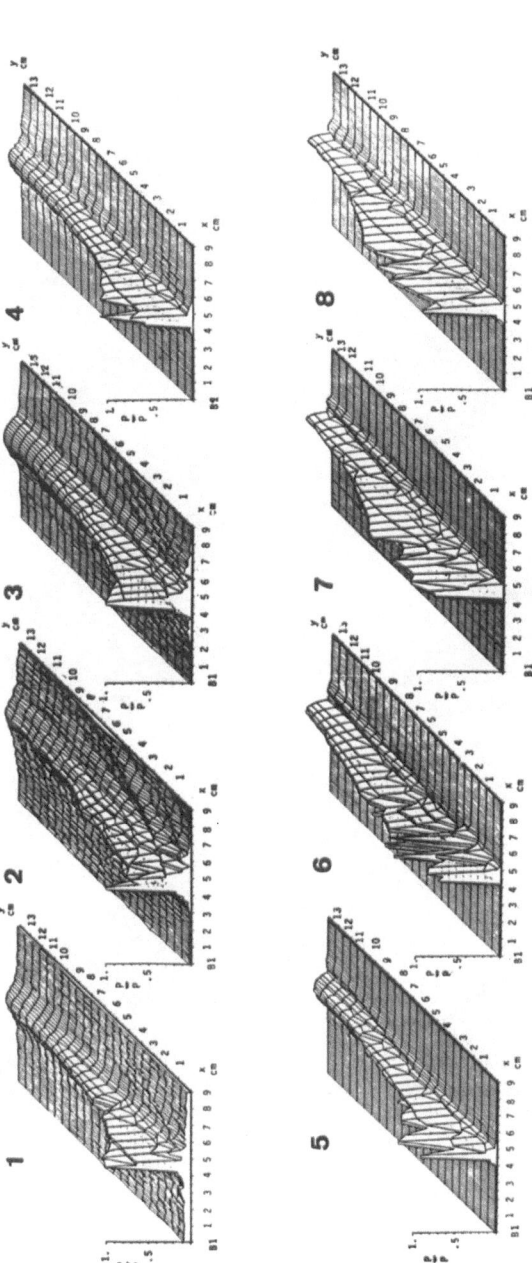

Fig. 4. Sound pressure distribution in a plane through the sound beam axis for a broad-band transducer. The diagrams are normed by their maxima, the parameter is the frequency of the input signal in MHz.

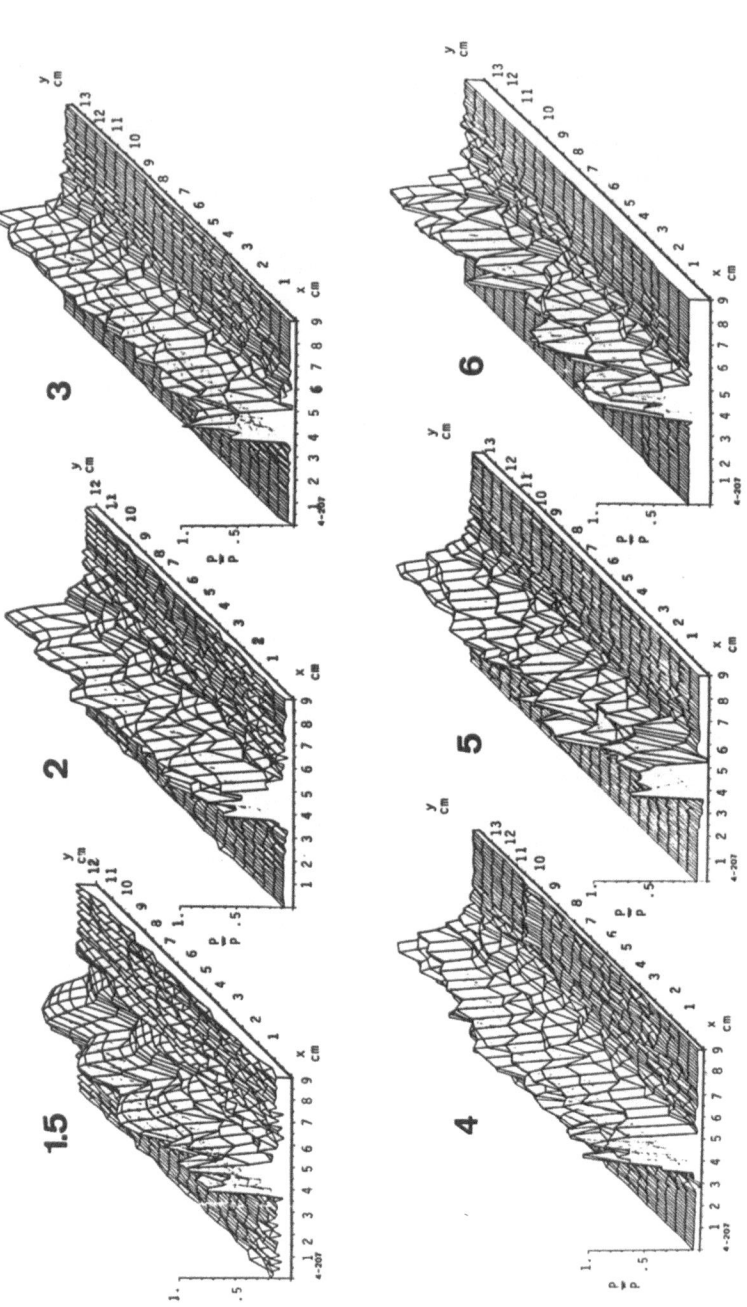

Fig. 5. Sound pressure distribution in a plane through the sound beam axis for a 4 MHz small band transducer. The diagrams are normed by their maxima, the parameter is the frequency of the input signal in MHz.

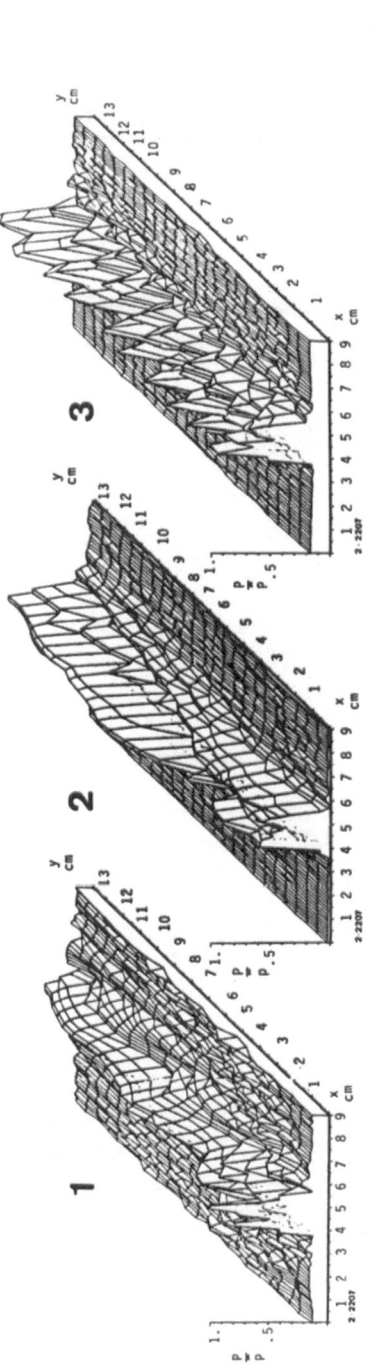

Fig. 6.   Sound pressure distribution in a plane through the sound beam axis for a 2 MHz small band transducer.   The diagrams are normed by their maxima, the parameter is the frequency of the input signal in MHz.

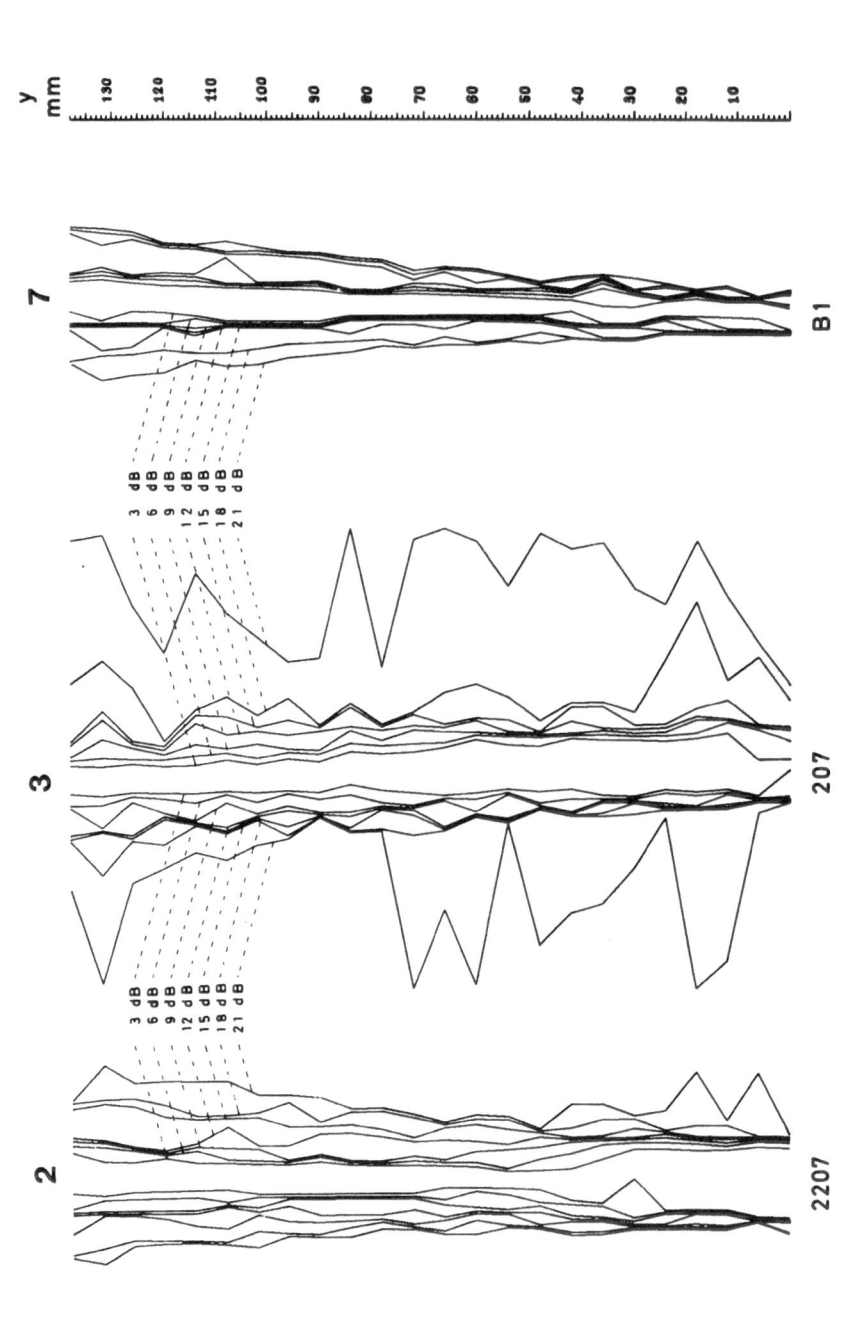

Fig. 7. Range dependent relative pressure decreases of characteristic lobes of Figs. 5., 6. and 7. The scale applies in all directions.

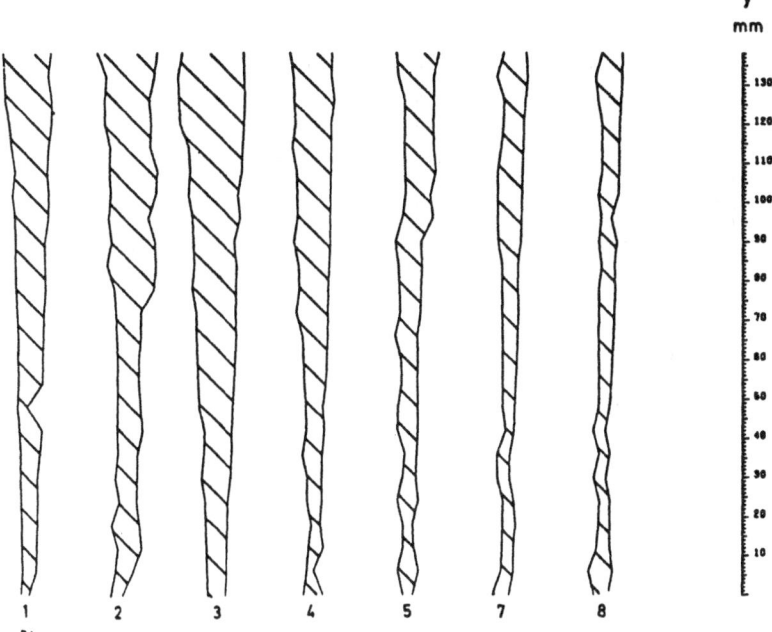

Fig. 8. Dependence of the 3 dB-main lobe on the excitation frequency
         for the broad-band transducer.

To determine the frequency dependence of the transmitters the
radiation force method and cw-excitation were used[3]. Fig. 9.
shows the results for the three transducers discussed. The
3 dB-bandwidth could be determined by these measurements to be
3.75 MHz for the broad-band transducer and 1.67 MHz and 0.5 MHz
for the 4 MHz and 2 MHz small band transducers, respectively.

SUMMARY

    A broad-band transducer with two $\lambda/4$-matching layers is
presented, which was specially developed for medical ultrasonic
spectroscopy. By extensive measurements of transmitter characteristics, the spatial dependence on spectral composition of the
transmitted signal, as well as of sound beam profiles as a function
of range and excitation frequency, were investigated. The results
are compared with those from commercial transducers.

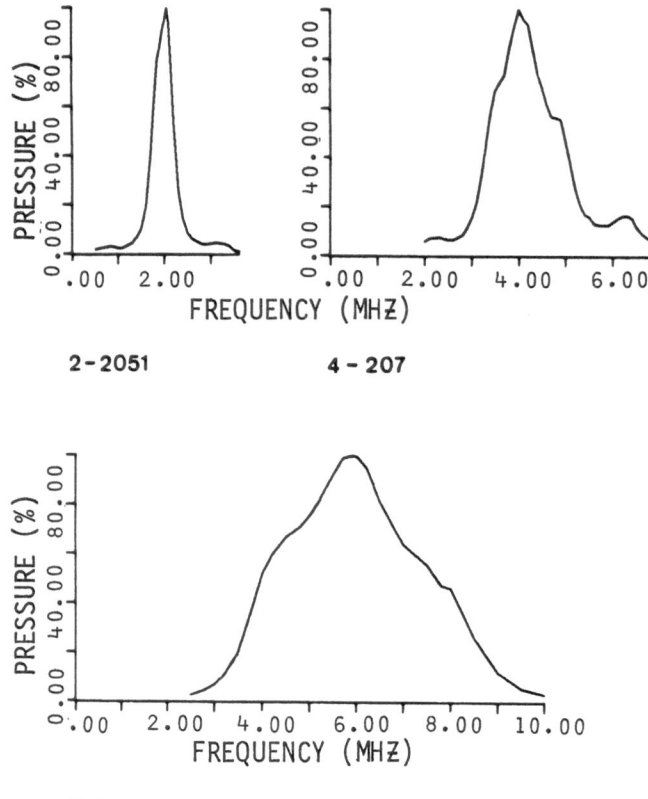

Fig. 9. Frequency dependence on the emitted spatial and time
         averaged power of 2 and 4 MHz small band transducers, as
         well as of the broad-band transducer.

REFERENCES

1. K.-P. Richter, R. Millner and I. Danz, Properties of ultrasonic
    broad-band transducers with a multilayer matching to water,
    in: "Proceedings FASE 78", Warsaw (1978), p.322-324.
2. N. Leitgeb and S. Schuy, Grenzflächendifferenzierung durch
    Raumwinkel-Scannen, in: "Ultraschalldiagnostik", Georg Thieme
    Verlag, Stuttgart (1978), p.17-20.
3. P. Wach, F. Holzer and N. Leitgeb, Über eine Anwendung der
    Schallstrahlungsdruck-Methode zur Messung der von einem
    Ultraschall-Diagnostikgerät abgegebenen Schalleistung, in:
    "Proceedings 4. Jahrestagung der Österr. Ges. f. Biomed.
    Technik, Graz (1979), p.73-77.

NUMERICAL CALCULATION OF NEARFIELD PRESSURE VARIATIONS OF DIFFERENT ANNULAR RING TRANSDUCERS

B. Gassman, K.-P. Richter and R. Millner

Institute of Applied Biophysics
Martin-Luther-University
DDR-4041 Halle, Strasse der DSF 81, GDR

INTRODUCTION

The medical ultrasonic diagnosis calls for ultrasonic transducers with a better spatial resolution. Computer modeling of the sound-fields was a useful help in transducer design. The computations of soundfields was based on the RAYLEIGH-integral[1]. Due to the solution method of this integral, the nearfield of FRESNEL-zone and the farfield or FRAUNHOFER-zone must be distinguished. The farfield approximation can be computed analytically. The calculation of the nearfield is a numerical approximation of the integral[2]. Today high speed methods are used for the approximation of soundfields [3, 4]. These methods based on a convenient transformation of the differential equation second order of a linear system into a differential equation first order. The solution of this equation is called the impulse-response-function (IRF). The IRF of a circular piston source is known, and the soundfields of circular piston and circular ring transducers were computed. Also the diffraction loss curves of these transducers were calculated[5, 6].

METHODS

The calculation of the pressure variations of a transducer in continuous wave excitation were based on the RAYLEIGH-integral

$$p = \frac{i\rho c}{\lambda} e^{i\omega t} \int_F V(x_1 \; x_2) \frac{e^{-ikr}}{r} \, dF$$

Using the impulse-response-method only a simple integration is necessary, but the RAYLEIGH-integral requires a summation of the area elements of the whole transducer. The advantage of the IRF method is the high speed of calculation.

The RAYLEIGH-integral changes to the following expression if a piston source is considered[3]

$$p = i\omega\rho V_o \ e^{i\omega t} \int_{-\infty}^{\infty} h(x,\tau)e^{-i\omega r} \ dr$$

where ρ   density
      c   velocity
      λ   wavelength
      ω   circular frequency
   V, V_o velocity amplitude
      r   distance between dF and the fieldpoint
      τ   transmission time
      F   area
      t   time

Calculations of circular piston and circular ring transducers were carried out. Based on the impulse-response for circular pistons the impulse-response for circular ring pistons was pointed out. The coordinate system shown in Fig. 1. was used.

Z means the distance of a fieldpoint in front of the transducer area. R_1 and R_2 indicate the two cases of possible projections $L(R_1)$

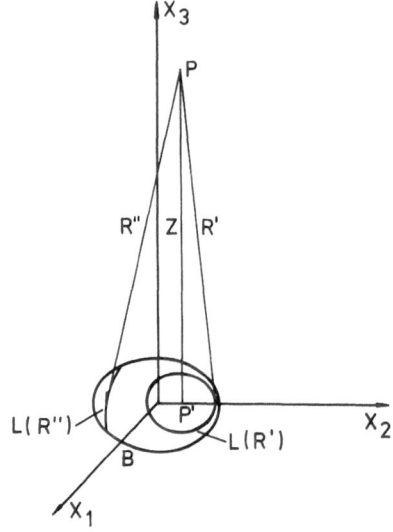

Fig. 1.   Coordinate system for the impulse-response calculation.

and $L(R_2)$, with

$$R_1 = (z^2+(r-B)^2)^{1/2} ,$$

and

$$R_2 = (z^2+(r+B)^2)^{1/2} .$$

The impulse-response depends on the expression R=ct. It has a constant value e.g.

$$h(r,z,t) = 0$$

or

$$h(r,z,t) = c$$

or is an arcos-function e.g.

$$h(r,z,t) = c/\pi \ arcos \left\{ \frac{(ct)^2-z^2+r^2-B^2}{2r((ct)^2-z^2)^{1/2}} \right\}$$

where B   transducer radius
      r   distance of the fieldpoint from the acoustical axis
    R=ct space-time-equivalence

If a circular ring transducer is considered, three cases must be distinguished:

A< (B−A)/2
A= (B−A)/2
A> (B−A)/2

Thereby the projection of the fieldpoint may be within the internal circle, between the internal and the external circle or outside of the transducer area, shown in Fig. 2. The boundary conditions are given by the arc of:

$$R_1 = (z^2+(r-A)^2)^{1/2}$$

$$R_2 = (z^2+(r+A)^2)^{1/2}$$

$$R_3 = (z^2+(r-B)^2)^{1/2}$$

$$R_4 = (z^2+(r+B)^2)^{1/2} .$$

The impulse-response is a constant e.g.

$$h(r,z,t) = c$$

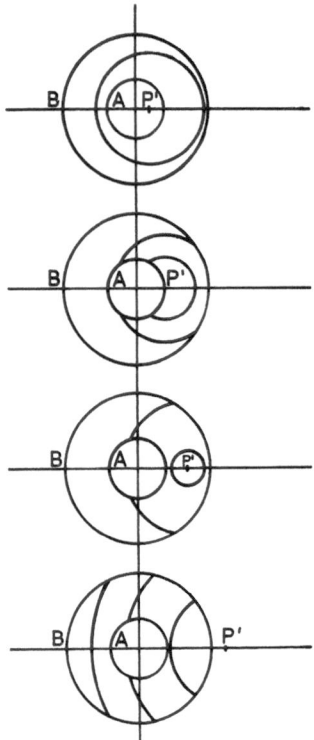

Fig. 2.   Projections on the ring transducer.
A - inside radius   B - outside radius

or a combination of the functions

$$IRF(A) = c/\pi \; \arccos \left\{ \frac{R^2-z^2+r^2-A^2}{2r(R^2-z^2)^{1/2}} \right\}$$

and

$$IRF(B) = c/\pi \; \arccos \left\{ \frac{R^2-z^2+r^2-B^2}{2r(R^2-z^2)^{1/2}} \right\} ,$$

depending on the expression R=ct.

RESULTS

The soundfields of circular ring transducers with the same outside radius but diverse inside radii and the same radiated wavelength
were calculated. Three-dimensional models of the calculated soundfields were designed. The magnitude is given by the amount of the

complex sound pressure. The acoustical and radial axes were
normalized. Figs. 3., 4. and 5. show the nearfield of circular
and circular ring pistons, where A is the inside radius, B the outside
radius and λ the wavelength.

Also the diffraction loss curves were calculated. Three cases
of the receiving transducer were considered. On the one hand the ring
transducer itself acts as receiver and on the other the inner
transducer with the radius A or the inner and the ring transducer
act as receiver. Figs. 6. and 7. show the behavior of different
transducers.

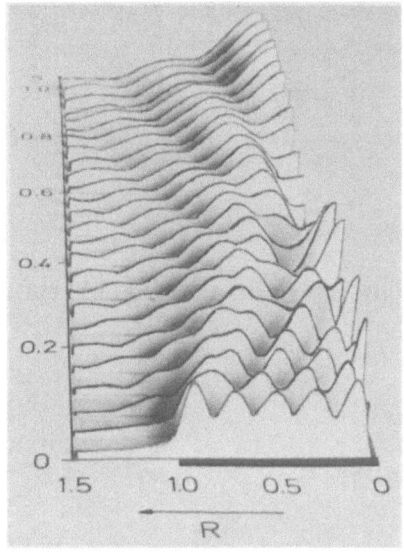

Fig. 3. Soundfield of circular piston, B/λ = 5.

DISCUSSION

The effect of different central bores of ring transducers on
the soundfield were investigated. A focusing effect is clearly
seen, but the number of the side lobes increase with the diameter
of the central bore. The diffraction loss curves also showed the
focusing effect of this type of transducer.

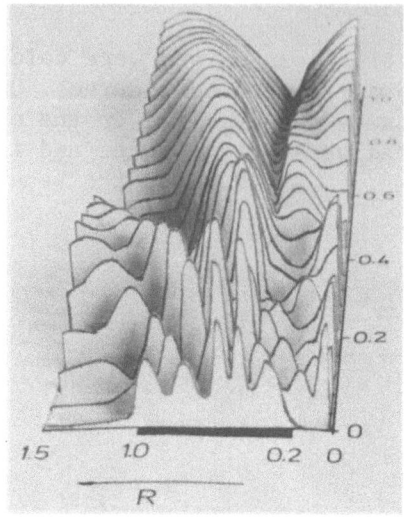

Fig. 4.　Soundfield of a circular ring piston,　B/λ = 5, A/λ = 1.

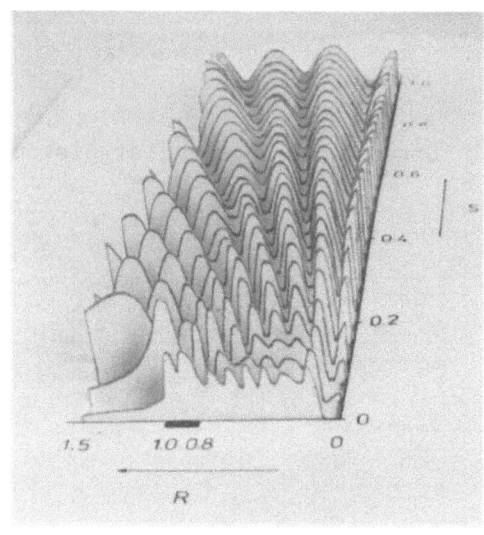

Fig. 5.　Soundfield of a circular ring piston,　B/λ = 5, A/λ = 4.

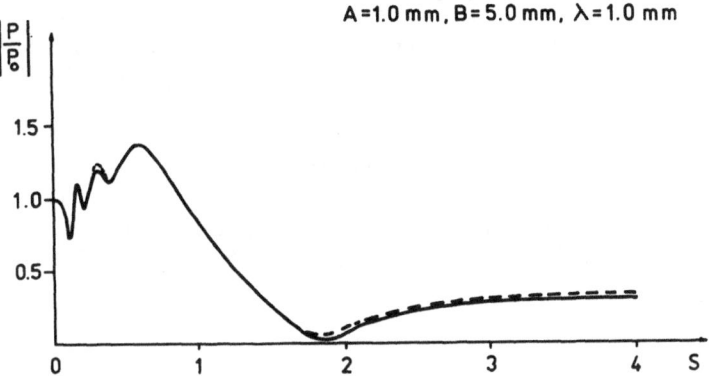

Fig. 6.   Diffraction loss of a ring transducer.

―――――― receiver – ring transducer
------ receiver – whole transducer

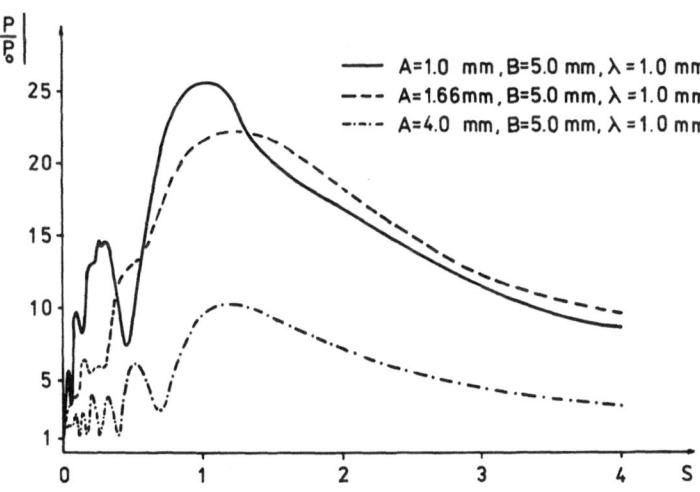

Fig. 7.   Diffraction loss of different ring transducers with the
          inner circular transducer as receiver.

REFERENCES

1. J. W. S. Rayleigh, "Theory of Sound", Dover Publ., New York (1945).
2. J. Zemanek, Beam behavior within the nearfield of a vibrating
    piston, J. Acoust. Soc. Am. 49:181-191 (1971).
3. J. C. Lockwood and J. G. Wilette, High speed method for computing
    the exact solution for the pressure variations in the nearfield
    of a baffled piston, J. Acoust. Soc. Am. 53:735-741 (1973).
4. P. Stepanishen, Asymptotic behavior of the acoustic nearfield of
    a circular piston, J. Acoust. Soc. Am. 59:749-754 (1976).
5. K. Brendel and G. Ludwig, Measurement of diffraction loss for
    circular transducers, Acustica 32:110-113 (1975).
6. B. Fay, Numerische Berechnung der Beugungsverluste im Schallfeld
    von Ultraschallwandlern, Acustica 36:209-213 (1976/1977).

MODEL FOR THE CALCULATION OF SENSITIVITY ULTRASONIC DOPPLER TRANSDUCERS

U. Cobet and H. J. Münch

Institute of Applied Biophysics
Martin-Luther-University Halle
DDR-4014 Halle, Strasse der DSF 81, GDR

Theoretical estimations and experimental examinations on the sensitivity of continuous wave ultrasonic Doppler transducers show that both the acoustics as well as the electric matching have a considerable influence on the sensitivity of transducer systems. That is why model calculations are being carried out. In the case of coupled transducers we must assume that ideally there has to be a smooth piston action. The calculations are simplified by the fact that with a continuous wave operation, we only need to take the steady-state condition into consideration. Nevertheless the internal absorption of probe material and matching layers have a considerable influence.

It can be shown, based on the theory of Mason[1] and the calculations of Kossoff et al.[2] that when a plane sound wave passes a layer, the four-terminal network theory can also be used if this layer has internal absorption (Fig. 1.). The wave comes from an absorbing, semi-infinite space and penetrates into a space with the same features. Thus, the idea of emitting into a space is only to be realized if there is an internal absorption of a relatively great amount. Then, if the input potential is double and as usual the input impedance of semi-infinite space is put in series and the output impedance parallel, we obtain exact results.

A modified six-terminal network according to Mason[1] was used as an equivalent circuit for the transducer (Fig. 2.). The results show that the sensitivity is influenced by the internal absorption of the piezoelectric material. Therefore the sound attenuation was again taken into account in the equivalent circuit by introducing a complex transfer function γ.

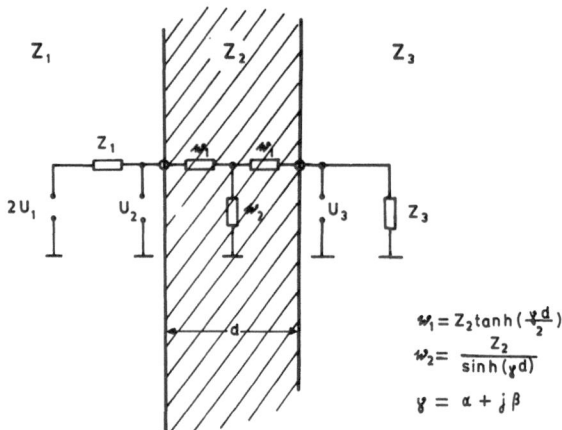

Fig. 1. Equivalent circuit for acoustic matching layer with

  Z_i the acoustic impedance of material i
  α the attenuation

$\beta = \dfrac{2\pi}{\lambda_2}$ the phase shift

  λ_2 the wavelength of material 2

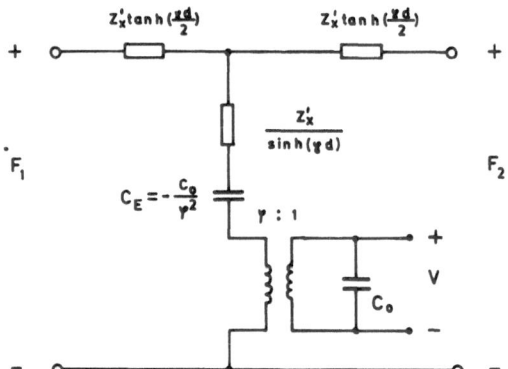

Fig. 2. Modified equivalent circuit of a thickness mode transducer
         from Mason[1] with C_o as the clamped capacity, $Z_x = Z_x A$
         with A as the area of the transducer and ϕ the ideal
         transformation ratio, by using the analogy force F to
         voltage V.

The resistance of the symmetric T-network, which shall characterize the acoustic features of the probe, were replaced by sinh (γd) and tanh ($\frac{\gamma d}{2}$).

Because piezoelectrical ceramics have a relatively high electro-acoustic coupling factor the electric side has a significant reaction, which is not to be neglected, on the acoustic side and vice versa. These interconnections are very complex. Therefore a simple FORTRAN program was used. Due to the internal absorption there were no poles.

Fig. 3. is the complete equivalent circuit of the transmitting system. The following were taken into account:

- the dynamic features of the piezoelectric probe
- a maximum of 2 acoustic matching layers to the tissue
- a backward acoustic layer which acts as the coupling vibrator and energy store and -- if it is necessary -- a frequency adjustment is possible
- a compensation of the clamped capacity of the probe by a coil, which acts as a parallel resonant circuit with a special Q-factor
- a matching to the electric cable
- the reaction of the electric cable itself
- the input and output resistance of the device.

Analogous for the transmitter system, Fig. 4. is the complete equivalent circuit of the receiving system, however, after having been transformed on the acoustic side. Again, the internal absorption of the materials was taken into account.

Now the typical behavior will be shown by means of some calculation examples performed on 5 MHz transducers of Piezolan S and Piezolan S2 which have a diameter of 10 mm from the ceramic factory Hermsdorf. In Fig. 5. the sensitivity of the transmitting and receiving system is plotted against the frequency. There is a direct acoustic coupling to the tissue without matching layers and an electrical matching only with a transmitting output of low resistance and a receiving input of high resistance. The internal absorption of the probe is very small and the backing material is air. Due to the clamped capacity there is a characteristic shift of the frequency between the maximum sensitivity of the transmitting and receiving system, of about 300 kHz.

A ceramic with a high transformation ratio such as Piezolan S2 makes a good transmitter, whereas a ceramic with a low transformation ratio, for example, Piezolan S, is useful to increase the sensitivity of a receiver. Compared to this the sensitivity of a ceramic with a relatively low Q-factor of 50 is plotted. You can see that the maximum sensitivity is decreased by about 3 to 4 dB for both the receiver and transmitter.

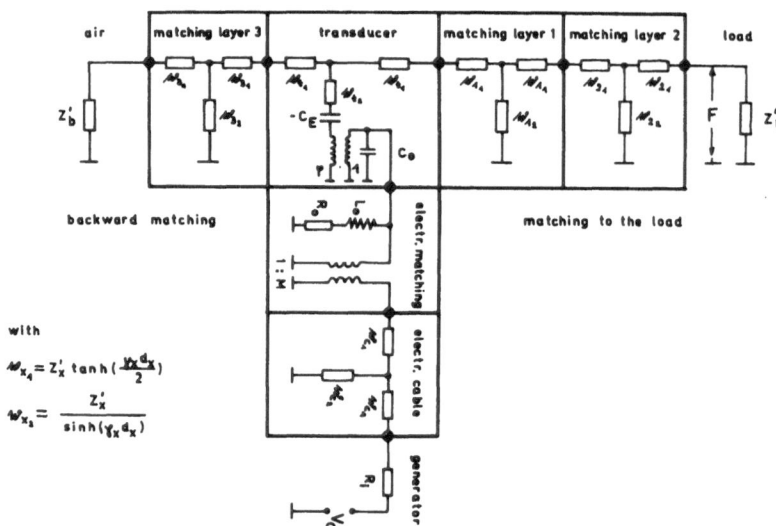

Fig. 3.   Equivalent circuit for the transmitting transducer.

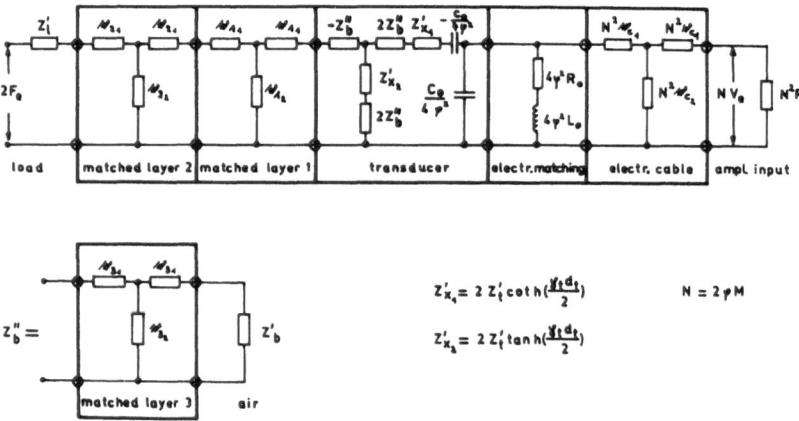

Fig. 4.   Simplified equivalent circuit for the receiving transducer.

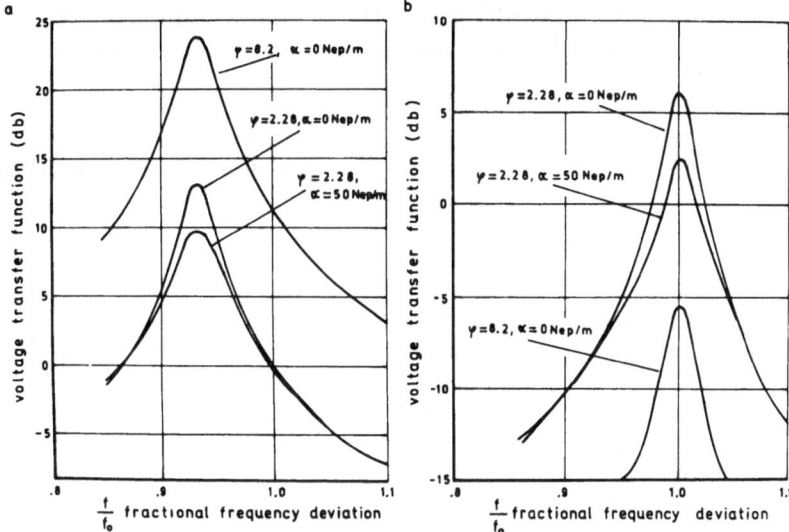

Fig. 5. Voltage transfer function of the transmitting (a) and
receiving (b) system to the frequency for Piezolan S2 with
$\phi = 8.2$ and Piezolan S with $\phi = 2.28$.

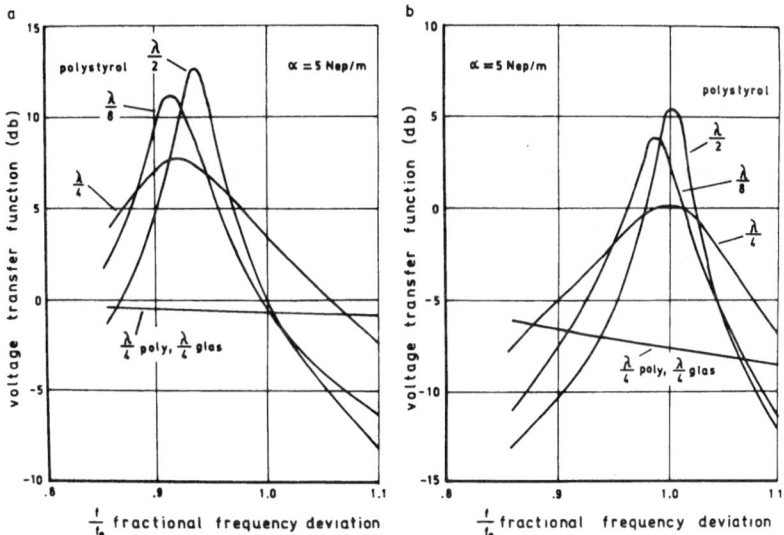

Fig. 6. Voltage transfer function of a transmitting (a) and
receiving (b) transducer to the frequency for matching
layers to the load.

In order to protect the transducer from damage and to make it suitable for acoustic matching to the tissue, coupling layers are frequently used. In Fig. 6. the sensitivity of a transmitting and receiving system is shown which has matching layers consisting of polystyrol with dimensions a quarter wave and a half wave. Although an improved acoustic matching can be achieved by a quarter wave matching layer, the sensitivity decreases due to higher damping.

SUMMARY

The model calculations have shown that especially the sensitivity of the transmitting system is decreased, if an electric cable is used without special coupling to it. In addition to this, it is obvious that on the one hand a frequency adjustment can be performed and on the other hand the Q-factor, and hence the sensitivity, can be increased by using a suitable, backward matching layer. But this is always connected with a higher degree of effort to produce such transducers.

Furthermore, the model calculations indicate that the sensitivity of cw-Doppler transducers can be improved by using an asymmetric construction, that means a separate optimum transmitting and receiving system.

REFERENCES

1. W. P. Mason, "Physical Acoustics", Academic Press, New York,
       San Francisco, London (1964), Volume 1, Part 1.
2. G. Kossoff, D. E. Robinson and W. J. Garrett, The Cal Abdominal
       Echoscope, in: "Commonwealth Acoustic Laboratories Report
       No. 31", Sydney, Australia (1965).

REVIEW OF THE PHYSICAL BASES FOR BIOLOGICAL TISSUE CHARACTERIZATION

BY ULTRASOUND

M. Hussey, A. Moore and J. Callis *

Dublin Institute of Technology, Kevin Street,
Dublin 8, Ireland, and Irish Foundation for Human
Development, St. James' Hospital, Dublin 8, Ireland

Imaging of tissues by means of ultrasound is now a vital element in the diagnostic armoury of medicine. In the development of the requisite equipment, the foundation stone has been the understanding of the modes of interaction between ultrasound and biological tissues [1]. Furthermore, there has been a dynamic interplay between the extent of this understanding and the diagnostic technology. Advances on one front have served to spur advances on the other.

The present phase of this process consists of the many efforts to derive specific ultrasound characteristics for the different tissue types. Ultimately it is envisaged that histology and pathology may be achieved in vivo. The other side of this process is the introduction of digital signal processing techniques into the diagnostic equipment. In this paper it is proposed to examine the evolution of this interplay between our understanding of the interaction mechanisms and the performance of the clinical diagnostic equipment.

ULTRASOUND TISSUE MODEL MARK I

The first generation of ultrasound imaging devices were the bistable B-mode scanning units. In these instruments, the pulsed ultrasound beam interrogates a slab of tissue and produces a cross-sectional view of that slab in which the outlines of the organs -- in effect the large acoustic interfaces within the slab -- are displayed

*The authors wish to thank the Leverhulme Trust Fund, the Cancer Research Advancement Board of the Irish Cancer Society and the Irish Foundation for Human Development for supporting this work.

in correct geometrical relationship to each other. Basically specularly reflecting surfaces of sufficient extent are imaged. The
continuum of the tissue enveloped by these surfaces is neglected,
except in so far as it possesses an intrinsic constant speed of
propagation, c, and acoustic impedance, Z, and an attenuation
coefficient, $\alpha^{(2,3,4)}$.

The speed of propagation given by

$$c = \sqrt{K/\rho} \; ,$$

where K is the tissue bulk modulus and ρ is its density, determines
the pulse echo return time and so the relative positioning of the
echoes on the image. It is effectively independent of frequency in
soft tissues in the diagnostic range of frequencies. Also its value
for most soft tissues is very close to the value for water, as
indicated in Table 1. The characteristic acoustic impedance given by

$$Z = \rho c \; ,$$

Table 1. Approximate values of propagation
speed, c(ms), characteristic acoustic
impedance, $Z(10^6 kg/m^2 s)$, and
attenuation coefficient, α(dB/cm), for
some tissues at 1MHz at 37°C.

Tissue	c	Z	α
water	1510	1.51	-
blood	1560	1.56	.09
fat	1460	1.39	.6
brain	1520	1.57	.9
nerve	1610	1.68	.9
liver	1570	1.65	.9
kidney	1560	1.64	.9
muscle	1630	1.73	3.5
lung	650	.26	41.0
lens	1620	1.84	2.5
bone	3050	5.0	8.7

helps to determine the reflection coefficients at different boundaries and hence the echo signal strengths. But in the bistable display, the range of echo amplitudes is of no consequence provided they are above the minimum threshold level set by the suppressor.

In combination, the speed of propagation and the characteristic acoustic impedance values provide the design data for constructing depends on the degree of mismatch, on the shape of the scatterer on its size relative to the ultrasound wavelength. Fig. 3. shows the scattering behavior at a spherical inhomogeneity of radius a. Some salient points should be noted about this behavior. At low frequencies, the scattering is slight and is mostly backscattering contained in a solid angle directed back towards the source transducer. At higher frequencies, there is much more power scattered but most of it is diffracted downstream along the z-axis, while a small amount is backscattered as before.

Other scatterer shapes could be expected to yield other fine-detailed behavior, but the general frequency or wavelength dependence would be similar.

The internal microstructure of tissues may be viewed as ensembles of such scatterers -- the fibrillar structure of muscle, the lobular structure of the liver, etc. Therefore the complex of scattering phenomena in an ultrasound beam would occur at many sites in a wide range of phase relationships. The loss of power out of the beam results in bulk attenuation which rises with frequency and which acts in conjunction with the attenuation due to relaxational absorption as indicated in Fig. 4., to yield the total overall attenuation. Very likely the differences in total attenuation coefficients between tissue types are mostly due to the scattering moiety, which in turn is a reflection of the microstructural differences between the tissue types.

The pulse echo interrogation of these tissues allows of the reception of the backscattered echoes by the transducer. But since the scatterers have a variety of sizes and are located at a variety of ranges from the transducer, the received backscattered echo signal the bistable instrument.

The attenuation coefficient of the tissues enters as a complicating factor. It reduces the strength of the echoes, producing a greater reduction for the "deeper" echoes. Normally this is compensated for by means of the depth gain compensation function of the instrument, but because as shown in Table 1., different tissues have different values of attenuation coefficient, compensation can only be approximate. One salient feature of the attenuation coefficient is its strong frequency dependence. Fig. 1. represents some of the data in this connection. Many results, such as those of Miller et al[5, 6], shown in Fig. 2., show that attenuation not only depends on tissue type but also on the state of the tissue.

The conceptual model of the tissues in the bistable technology is basically one of aqueous solutions characterized by different attenuation properties. This model emerged particularly from the common methods of measuring tissue properties -- the single pass transmission techniques which respond to the aggregate or bulk properties of the tissue sample place between the transmitting and receiving transducers.

At this bulk level, Table 1. shows that the attenuation coefficient of the tissues offers some clear means of distinguishing different tissue types. Data such as that shown in Fig. 3. offer the possibility that attenuation measurements might allow the characterization of disease conditions and pathology. Furthermore the frequency dependence of overall attenuation coefficient seems to present a usable basis for developing the details of characteristic indices for histologies and pathologies.

Unfortunately the conventional pulse echo technologies used in medical ultrasound imaging are not capable of yielding accurate measurements of tissue attenuation coefficient in vivo because of the complex geometries encountered in the body. Direct exploitation of this promising possibility awaits alternative technologies.

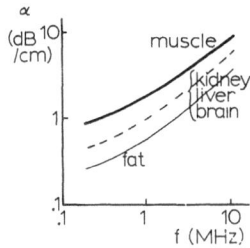

Fig. 1. Dependence of average attenuation coefficient on frequency
         for some tissues.

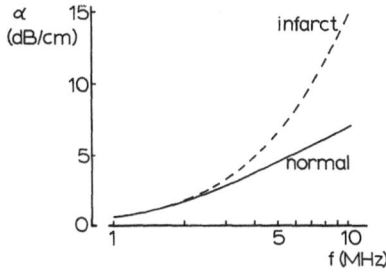

Fig. 2.   Frequency dependence of attenuation coefficient of myocardial
          muscle in healthy and infarcted state.

GREY SCALE IMAGING

     The advent of grey scale display techniques represented a major
step forward in medical ultrasound imaging. In this mode, weak
echo signals, previously rejected by the electronic processing in the
scanners, can be displayed with varying shades of grey between black
and white, depending on the signal strength. Not only are the smaller
specular reflectors displayed within the approximately 36 dB dynamic
range of these displays, but a new feature emerges, namely the
speckled pattern of greys within the bulk of the tissues. In
consequence, the acoustically homogeneous tissue model has to be
refined.

ULTRASOUND TISSUE MODEL MARK II

     Backscattering of the pulsed incident ultrasound from cells and
multicellular aggregates is invoked as the primary mechanism giving
rise to the intra-organ speckled patterns in the grey scale images.
Scattering occurs when the incident plane wave encounters a very
small inhomogeneity. The disturbance of the forward travelling wave

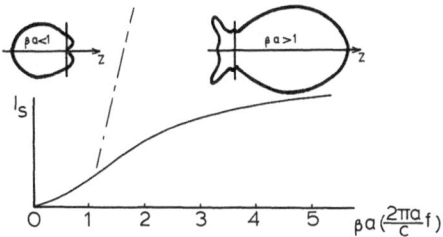

Fig. 3.   The frequency dependence of backscattered intensity I_s
          and the polar diagrams of the backscattering for different
          frequencies and scatterer radii.

from internal tissue microstructures consists of a complex interference signal. Thus at any instant, the pulse echo signal received
at a given delay, conventionally attributed to a fixed depth into the
tissue, is the instantaneous sum of the acoustic pressures of the
elemental echoes from a number of scattering centres, ranging in size,
depth and location across and along the beam. These scatterers
possibly also vary in composition and shape.

The nature, distribution and concentration of these acoustic
scatterers may be assumed to vary from one tissue to another and
from one pathological state to another. The Mark II ultrasound
tissue model as shown in Fig. 5. therefore emerges. Clearly a
detailed examination of the backscattering effected by various tissues
may be expected to yield useful diagnostic information about those
tissues and may even yield clear and unequivocal characterizations
of tissue state and health.

Such efforts occupy the minds of many researchers at the present
time[7,8,9]. One approach, being used by the present authors, is to
be discussed in a later paper[10].

ULTRASOUND TISSUE MODEL MARK III

There is one other noteworthy feature of tissues, which is
involved in their interactions with ultrasound, and which occurs in
vivo but not in vitro and did not enter into the earliest concepts
of the acoustic behavior of tissues. This is motion. Tissue
movement can arise due to a variety of causes such as proximity to
organs of motion such as the heart, diaphragm or other muscles, or
arterial pulsations due to blood flow. In conventional imaging such
motions are suppressed or minimized to prevent blurring, by having
the patient hold inspiration or by some other such measure. But the
advent of the advanced dynamic scanners allows the visualization of
the movement within organs and tissues. On the dynamic grey scale

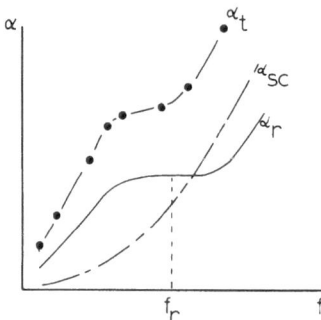

Fig. 4.   Relaxational absorption coefficient α_r is added to
          scattering attenuation coefficient α_{sc} to yield the total
          attenuation coefficient α_t.

image it manifests as a twinkling and sparkling of the normal speckled pattern. Such twinkling may be readily envisaged as arising from the oscillatory movements of the small scatterers within the tissues. These movements may quite likely be typical or characteristic of the organ in question and indeed of the location of the vibratory scatterers within the tissue. Study of the dynamic features of the backscattered echo signals, by time domain or doppler shift or other methods, may be expected to yield still more detailed specifications of tissues and indeed of even small regions within organs.

SUMMARY

The most up-to-date ultrasound model of tissues in vivo is one in which each tissue type is surrounded by a specularly reflecting outer membrane. The tissue interior consists of a three dimensional mosaic of scattering centers, engaged in some movement, embedded in an aqueous type medium. Study of and measurement of the dynamic backscattering from the tissue interiors seems to offer the best possibility for objectively characterizing the tissue histology and pathology by pulse echo ultrasound methods.

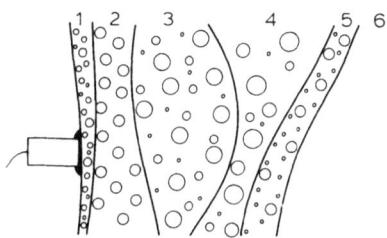

Fig. 5. Mark II ultrasound model of tissues with different
         distributions of scattering centres, of a variety of sizes,
         in different tissues.

REFERENCES

1. M. Hussey, "Diagnostic Ultrasound: An Introduction to the
    Interactions between Ultrasound and Biological Tissues",
    Blackie & Son, Ltd., Glasgow (1975).
2. S. A. Goss, R. L. Johnston and F. Dunn, Comprehensive compilation
    of empirical ultrasonic properties of mammalian tissues,
    J. Acoust. Soc. Am. 64:423 (1978).
3. S. A. Goss, R. L. Johnston and F. Dunn, Compilation of empirical
    ultrasonic properties of mammalian tissues II, J. Acoust. Soc.
    Am. 68:93 (1980).
4. R. C. Chivers and R. J. Parry, Ultrasonic velocity and attenu-
    ation in mammalian tissues, J. Acoust. Soc. Am. 63:940 (1978).
5. J. G. Miller et al., Ultrasonic tissue characterization: corre-
    lation between biochemical and ultrasonic indices of
    myocardial injury, in: "Proc. IEEE Ultrasonics Symposium,
    1976".
6. D. E. Yuhas et al., Changes in ultrasonic attenuation indicative
    of regional myocardial infarction, Ultrasound in Medicine 3
    (1977).
7. J. M. Thijssen, ed., "Ultrasonic Tissue Characterization:
    Clinical Achievements and Technological Potentials", Stafleu's
    Scientific Publishing Co., Brussels (1980).
8. M. deBilly and G. J. Quentin, Methods of analysis for back-
    scattering from tissues, Ultrasonics 85 (1979).
9. M. Linzer, ed., "Ultrasonic Tissue Characterization, I, II,
    III", National Bureau of Standards, Washington (1976, 1979,
    1980).
10. A. Moore, J. Callis and M. Hussey, Ultrasound tissue character-
    ization using statistical analysis of the R. F. echo pulses,
    (this symposium).

ULTRASOUND TISSUE CHARACTERIZATION USING STATISTICAL ANALYSIS OF THE R. F. ECHO PULSES

A. Moore, J. Callis and M. Hussey

Dublin Institute of Technology, Kevin Street
Dublin 8, Ireland and Irish Foundation for Human
Development, St. James' Hospital, Dublin 8, Ireland

In the grey scale ultrasound image, different tissues present as different speckled patterns of greys, whites and blacks. Interpretation of these patterns now rests largely on the experienced operator/observer. Such pattern-recognition is best performed while in the the process of patient scanning, with the possibility of reviewing neighboring cross-sectional images, and indeed acquiring images from alternative angles of approach.

Many approaches are being investigated in the effort to develop objective methods of characterizing human tissues in vivo[1-5]. However, no method has yet been found which is superior to the pattern-recognition by the eye and brain of an experienced observer on a good grey scale image of the tissue in question.

In an attempt to discover such an objective method of characterizing tissues, the present work is aimed at examining the echo signals from within the tissues -- the backscattered portion of the echo train -- at the R. F. stage in the signal processing. On the basis that the detection stage in the scanner as well as the image formation stage in the scan converter may introduce some degradation of the information in the echoes, the earlier in the signal processing path one analyzes the echoes the greater the likelihood of extracting tissue-specific information and hence the greater the chance of obtaining characteristic criteria.

The approach in this work is to sample the R. F. backscatter echo signals from a number of tissue types and to statistically analyze these sampled data by computer, in order to search for statistical indices to distinguish between the different tissues. Ultimately it is hoped to correlate any such indices with tissue

61

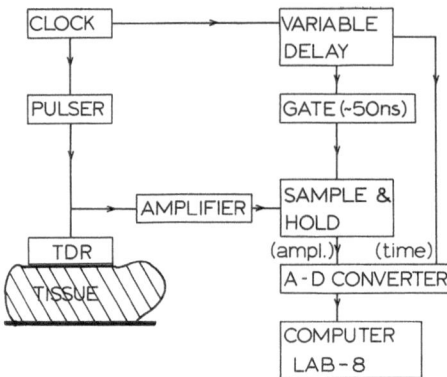

Fig. 1. Schematic diagram of the system used to digitize the back-
         scattered pulse echo signals from within tissue samples.

microstructure as well as with bulk acoustic properties of the tissues.

PROCEDURE

     Fig. 1. shows the system used in this work. The tissue slice
is coupled to a 2 MHz transducer by a coupling gel, all at room
temperature (~18°C). A Kretz Series 4150 MG A-mode unit is used to
stimulate the transducer. The same transducer was used in all the
studies reported here. In this way variations between transducers
and beam shapes were minimized. Any such variations due to the
nature of the path through the tissue traversed by the beam were
neglected at this stage.

     The received echo signals are first amplified and then sampled.
The sampling gate of 50 ns duration can be ranged manually from
0.2 cm to 1.3 cm along the beam axis, from the transducer face. At

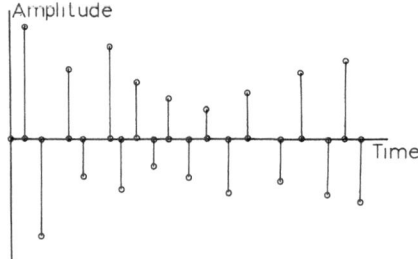

Fig. 2. Digitization of the peak and trough amplitudes and delays
         after the transmission pulse reduces the echo train to an
         array of impulses.

each setting of the gate, the amplitude and the time delay since the transmission pulse are digitized to 8 bits. The setting of the gate is chosen by monitoring the signal on an oscilloscope screen. In this work only the peaks and troughs are selected for digitizing. Each digitization is repeated 10 times and only the mean of these is stored in the computer memory. Effectively this process reduces the R. F. echo train to the array of impulse functions shown in Fig. 2.

For each specimen of tissue, some 10-15 echo signal trains are digitized in this way, yielding 10 or more arrays of data pairs for that specimen.

STATISTICAL ANALYSIS

The set of parameters listed in Table 1. are next derived from each array of data pairs. The mean ($\bar{x}$) and standard deviation (σ) of the values of each of these parameters are calculated. The salient features of the statistical distributions of these parameters are next quantified by calculation of the dispersion, skewness and kurtosis of each one. These latter quantities are defined thus.

$$\text{Dispersion} = \frac{\bar{x}}{\sigma} ,$$

$$\text{Skewness} = \frac{\sum_{i=1}^{n}\left(\frac{x_i-\bar{x}}{\sigma}\right)^3}{n} ,$$

$$\text{Kurtosis} = \frac{\sum_{i=1}^{n}\left(\frac{x_i-\bar{x}}{\sigma}\right)^4}{n} - 3 .$$

Table 1. List of the variables derived from each array of data pairs, to be used in the subsequent discriminant analysis.

Amplitudes of peaks
Amplitudes of troughs
Peak-trough amplitudes
Trough-peak amplitudes
Peak-peak amplitudes
Trough-trough amplitudes
Peak-peak delays
Trough-trough delays
Peak-trough slopes
Trough-peak slopes

Note that each of these distribution parameters is dimensionless. The dispersion is the normalized mean, the mean of an equivalent distribution in units of the standard deviation. The skewness of third moment of the distribution is a measure of the asymmetry of the actual distribution. It is zero for a normal distribution, positive for a distribution clustered lower than the mean and negative for a distribution with peak at a value higher than the mean. The kurtosis or fourth moment is a measure of how peaked or squat the actual distribution is. It is positive for a distribution more peaked than the normal, zero for the normal and negative for a distribution flatter than the normal.

These three dimensionless distribution parameters, for each of the 10 derived variables, constitute in all 30 parameters for each sample of tissue. These data are supplied to a DEC 20 mainframe computer for the discriminant analysis.

Similar data from all the tissue types shown in Table 2. were derived and served as the basic data for discriminant analysis by the commercially available SPSS package which has the appropriate subroutine called DISCRIMINANT.

The basic approach of this subroutine is to develop a linear combination of the 30 parameters (Z_j) for each tissue type, thus

$$D_i = d_{i,1}Z_1 + d_{i,2}Z_2 + \ldots\ldots d_{i,j}Z_j + \ldots\ldots + d_{i,30}Z_{30} \cdot$$

Here each $d_{i,j}$ is a weighting coefficient worked out by the program and D_i constitutes the score or value of the discriminant function i. In the ideal case the D scores for each array of data from specimens of the same type of tissue are identical. The task of the discriminant analysis program is to maximize the differences between D values for the different tissue types. The actual computer routine offers 6 sets of criteria whereby the weighting coefficients may be chosen for optimum discrimination. In general these methods first select the Z parameters that best differentiate the groups and thereafter other Z parameters are added into the linear combination, provided that they offer some minimum improvement in the discrimination.

Table 2.   Tissue types examined

Tissue	Code Number
Beef muscle	1
Lamb kidney	2
Lamb liver	3
Beef liver	4
Beef kidney	5

RESULTS

One of the simplest ways of displaying the discrimination
effected by the computer program is the scatter diagram, in which
the values of one D_i are plotted against another D_j, for the combined
data for each tissue specimen. Fig. 3. is such a plot. Note that
the data for each tissue specimen denoted by the relevant code numbers
result from at least 10 separate ultrasound beam traverses through the
tissue, sampled along approximately 1.2 cm of depth.

Clearly tissue type 5 is well separated from 3/4 and 1/2. The
latter two paired groups are also well differentiated from each other.
But types 3 and 4 overlap considerably even though their centroids,
denoted by the black circles, are clearly separated.

An alternative set of discriminant score pairs, plotted in
Fig. 4., offers a better differentiation between the five types of
tissue examined in this work.

The programme package has another element which estimates the
probability of an unknown tissue falling into any of the categories
1 - 5. Thus two sets of data measured "blind" were subjected to this
classification procedure. Table 3. shows the results of this.

SUMMARY

Clearly discrimant analysis can tease apart the data from the
five tissues examined in this work and can tentatively classify or
characterize data from an unknown one of these tissues. The program
can derive iso-probability contours around the centroid of each tissue
type group, so that the discriminant score D_i, for an unknown can
allow that tissue to be assigned with varying degrees of certainty
to one of the previously discriminated tissue types.

But it may well be necessary to obtain considerably more basic

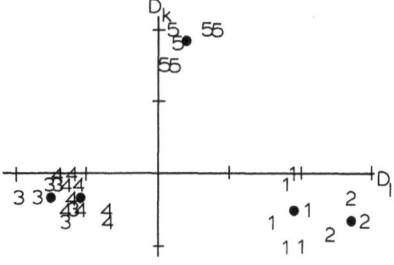

Fig. 3. A scatter diagram depicting two of the discriminant scores
         for all five types of tissue. Each code number represents
         one sample.

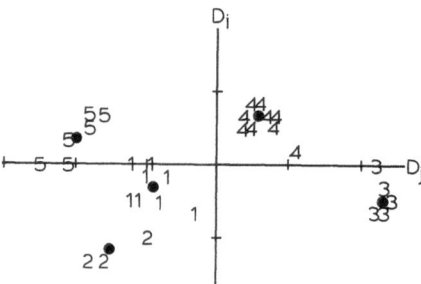

Fig. 4. An alternative scatter diagram, plotting two discriminant
scores other than those plotted in Fig. 3.

Table 3. Classification of data from "unknown" tissue

Actual group (X)	Highest probability group (G)	Estimated probability of X being in G	Second highest probability group (Y)	Estimated probability of X being in Y
1	1	.94	2	.02
4	4	.99	3	.002

data from many more tissue types, in order to more fully describe the
concentrations and distributions of data from the many different types
of tissue within the various regions of the scatter diagrams such as
Figs. 3. and 4.

Objective characterization of unknown data requires a large
data base from known tissue types, which will serve as the reference
or comparison library for future characterization tasks. The process
of gathering these data is now in progress. The job of comparing the
efficacy of this mode of characterization with the subjective methods
of pattern-recognition by an experienced observer reading the grey
scale image is still in the future.

REFERENCES

1. M. Linzer, ed., "Ultrasonic Tissue Characterization, I, II, III",
      National Bureau of Standards, Washington (1976, 1979 1980).
2. J. M. Thijssen, ed., "Ultrasonic Tissue Characterization:
      Clinical Achievements and Technological Potentials", Stafleu's
      Scientific Publishing Co., Brussels (1980).

3. M. deBilly and G. J. Quentin, Methods of analysis for backscattering from tissues, Ultrasonics 85 (1979).

4. M. Hussey, A. Moore and J. Callis, Review of the physical bases for biological tissue characterization by ultrasound, (this symposium).

5. K. Preston et al., Recent developments in obtaining histopathological information from ultrasound tissue signatures, in: "Ultrasonic Tissue Characterization, II", M. Linzer, ed., National Bureau of Standards, Special Publication 525, Washington (1979), p.303-312.

ACKNOWLEDGMENTS

The authors wish to thank the Leverhulme Trust Fund and the Cancer Research Advancement Board of the Irish Cancer Society for supporting this work.

MODELLING OF ULTRASONIC BACKSCATTERING FROM DISCRETE RANDOM SCATTERERS

I. Koch*

GEC Hirst Research Centre
Wembley
England

ABSTRACT

A comprehensive model of the scattering of ultrasound is used to calculate the backscattered pressure from two-dimensional arrays of cylindrical scatterers approximating the structure of muscle tissue.

Regular arrays of identical scatterers and random arrays of scatterers varying only in their radii are treated. First attempts at simple data analysis for these cases are described.

One of the effects of muscular dystrophy is a change in the propagation velocity of sound in the muscle cells. To model this situation, arrays of scatterers with different propagation velocities are considered and it is shown that even a small change in the velocities for muscle can change the echo pattern considerably.

INTRODUCTION

An increasing interest in the use of ultrasound in medical diagnostics has developed over the last decade, and different methods of characterizing tissue types have been tried. Most of the earlier techniques are of empirical nature and depend heavily on the equipment and the clinician's experience. To overcome these limitations, a more general knowledge of the physical interaction of ultrasound with tissue is needed.

---

*Now at: Department of Bio-Medical Physics, University of Aberdeen

Scattering from isotropic scatterers has been considered in the literature[e.g. 1,3,4,7]. In contrast to these approaches, we are interested in a better understanding of the physics of backscattering from non-isotropic scatterers using ultrasound.

We aim at characterizing muscle tissue which has a fairly regular, cylindrical structure. We apply our model of ultrasonic backscattering[5], which proved reliable for simple cylindrical scatterers, to random arrays of scatterers and we also examine elastic properties of the scatterers which are different for normal and diseased tissue.

DESCRIPTION OF THE MODEL

This is a brief summary of our scattering model. A more detailed version can be found in reference [5]. In a waterbath experiment, the amplitude of backscattered R. F. pulses is measured. The swept frequency R. F. is gated with variable gate width (1-9/us) and pulse repetition frequency (0.5-4 KHz). Typically, these echoes are from eleven nylon monofilaments placed 100 mm from a broad-band disc transducer.

In constructing a model of this experimental situation, the following were taken into account:

(a) beamprofile and "effective" transducer radius, which is about 10-13% smaller than the measured one,

(b) directivity of the disc transducer (first order Bessel function),

(c) spherical wave propagation restricted to the main lobe of the beam,

(d) transducer response,

(e) sampling volume, a function of beamwidth and beamlength-

The model is based on the inhomogeneous acoustic wave equation (e.g. [6]), and the backscattered pressure is the sum of the contributions from N scatterers.

$$p_s(\underline{r}_o) = \sum_{i=1}^{N} \int_V dV \left[k^2 \gamma_\kappa p G_{\underline{r}_o} - \nabla(\gamma_\rho \, \text{grad} p) \, G_{\underline{r}_o} \right] \qquad (1)$$

The pressure field p inside the scatterers is replaced by Born's incident field, and p also takes into account the above mentioned features, i.e.

$$p_i(\underline{r}) = \frac{a^2}{\lambda|\underline{r}|} \exp(ik|\underline{r}|) \, \frac{2J_1(ka\sin\phi)}{ka\sin\phi} \qquad (2)$$

ϕ as in Fig. 1., J_1 the first order Bessel function and G_r the Green's function. γ_K and γ_ρ are ratios of compressibilities and densities respectively.

In the case of the waterbath experiment, all scatterers had the same constant elastic properties. The experimental and theoretical pressure spectra showed good agreement.

BACKSCATTERING FROM RANDOM ARRAYS

First regular arrays of cylindrical point scatterers of the dimension of fibres, the cells of the muscle, were considered, but for the frequency range 4-8 MHz, the resolution was not adequate to separate the individual scatterers. Thus we concentrated on arrays of the dimension of muscle fasciculi (o.6-1.6 mm diameter) which can sometimes be resolved on B-scans. Regular rectangular arrays where rows and columns are separated by 1 mm, and hexagonal arrays of 1 mm spacing between neighbors were considered. The scattering target could be rotated about its center point and consisted of about 90-180 individual scatterers. For a fixed angle of rotation, θ (cf. Fig. 1.) varying from 0° to 45°, the backscattered pressure was calculated as a function of frequency and the whole cylindrical volume was taken into account. The obtained pressure spectra showed detailed structure arising from the individual scatterers. Since the fasciculi in a muscle are not regularly arranged one is interested to see how the echoes change when a local perturbation is introduced in the position of the scatterers. The position of the individual scatterers in the rectangular and hexagonal arrays was randomly varied, and the radii were changed accordingly. For a fixed angle, the pressure spectra of the regular and random arrays were compared, and it was noticed that even for the smallest deviation in the position of the scatterers, the pressure spectrum of the random array bears no resemblance to that of the regular array.

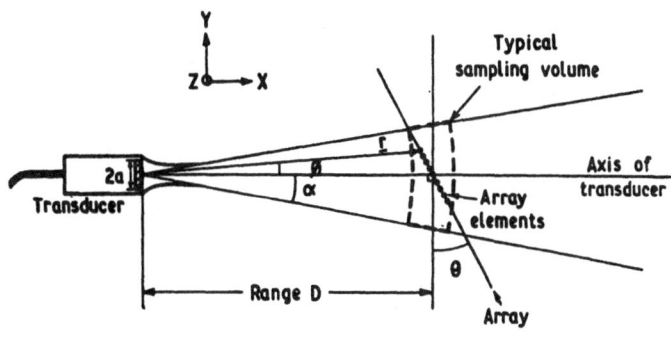

Fig. 1.

Due to the geometry of the regular hexagonal array, rotations by 0°, 60°, 120° etc. have the same pressure spectrum. Those angles θ with the same echo in the regular array, will be referred to as equivalent angles. We now compare the pressure spectrum for the 0° angle of the regular hexagonal array with the average over all 0-equivalent angles in the random array, and similarly for all angles between 0° and 30°. The result of these comparisons shows that, for all angles considered, the main peak in the spectrum is preserved in its frequency position and so also are some of the subsequent peaks. Thus averaging restores some of the symmetry lost in the individual random arrays, see Fig. 2.

DATA ANALYSIS AND PROCESSING

Autocorrelations in the Time Domain

The autocorrelations of the F. T.'s of the pressure, p_s, give the delays of echoes from non-equidistant scatterers. For one row of scatterers, they proved to be a successful device for analyzing echoes. If one deals with more than one row of scatterers, the autocorrelations no longer pick up the separation between individual scatterers. Instead, one would hope to see the separation between planes of scatterers, by which we mean rows of scatterers which are, for a fixed angle, normal to the transducer axis. In the case of the rectangular array, the separation between planes was picked up for 0° and 45°, and there, the expected separation agreed well with the computed one. For angles with less symmetry, the planes are no longer so clear, as individual scatterers interfere destructively.

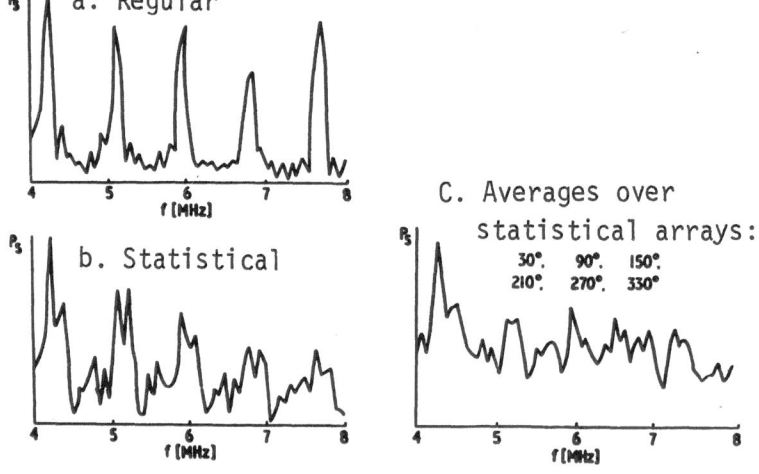

Fig. 2. Backscattered pressure from 30° hexagonal arrays.

For the hexagonal array, no echoes from planes could be seen at any angle in the autocorrelations. Thus, for two-dimensional arrays of scatterers, the autocorrelations in the time domain are no longer a sufficient device for analyzing the pressure spectrum.

Autocorrelation in the Frequency Domain

For discrete frequencies f_n varying from 4 to 8 MHz, one obtains autocorrelations over the discrete frequencies 0-4 MHz. From the first peak of f_p in this new spectrum, one wants to derive the mean separation $d = 0.5c/f_p$ between scatterers[2].

For the hexagonal array, the separation d at $0°$ and $30°$ indicated a separation in the direction normal to the transducer axis, rather than a spacing between scatterers. Averages over different angles of the same array give d = 1.03 mm in the hexagonal regular array corresponding well to the spacing of 1 mm between the scatterers, while d = 0.74 mm in the rectangular regular array reflects an average separation between the planes. For random arrays averaging was inconclusive.

Crosscorrelations in the Time Domain

For a given angle, the crosscorrelations were calculated for the spectra of the regular and random hexagonal arrays. The cross-correlations showed fewer peaks than the autocorrelation of the regular array at the same angle; but those peaks which did occur in the crosscorrelations agreed with peaks in the corresponding autocorrelations of the regular array.

One can also consider the crosscorrelations as a function of angle for a fixed time. We use t = 0, and are thus looking at the crosscorrelation coefficient. For the hexagonal arrays, the crosscorrelation coefficients were calculated for the following spectra:

(1) regular array at $0°$ with regular arrays varying over $360°$,

(2) regular array at $0°$ with random arrays varying over $360°$,

(3) random array at $0°$ with random arrays varying over $360°$.

The graph obtained from (1) is, of course, perfectly periodic, while the graph obtained from (3) shows very little periodicity, and the amplitudes are very much smaller than those in (1). In the graph obtained from (2), however, one can see that most of the peaks, expressing the periodicity in graph (1), are also present.

VELOCITY VARIATIONS AND COMPRESSIBILITY VARIATIONS

One of the distinguishing features between normal and diseased tissue is the change in the elastic properties. The propagation time c is related to the elastic constant κ, the compressibility, by $c^2 = (\kappa\rho)^{-1}$. Up to now we assumed a velocity of sound in water $c_o = 1.48 \times 10^6$ mm/s, and a constant velocity in the nylon scatterers, $c_1 = 2.68 \times 10^6$ mm/s. Now we want to consider different velocities inside the scatterers ranging from 1.585×10^6 mm/s (for muscle) to about 4×10^6 mm/s (for bone), and to look at the effects of random distributions of velocities about different means. For brevity we assume that the density remains constant, and only the compressibility changes as a result of velocity variations. Equation (1) can be split into two parts, containing only compressibility components and density components respectively. We now restrict ourselves to the part p_K of equation (1) which deals with the compressibility only.

$$p_K = \frac{\pi a^2}{\lambda^3} \sum_{i=1}^{N} I_i \gamma_{\kappa i} \quad \gamma_\kappa = \frac{\kappa_s - \kappa_o}{\kappa_o}$$

$I_i \gamma_{\kappa i}$ is the respective part of the integral in (1).

Since the velocity in the medium remains unchanged when the properties of the scatterers change, the following considerations will be based on c_o. c_1 will denote a constant velocity in the scatterers and $c_2 = \{c_{2i}\}$ $i = 1,\ldots,N$ will be the new velocities of the scatterers which are normally distributed about a mean. The following notation will be used; similarly for c and κ:

$$c_1 = c_o + \Delta_1 \qquad\qquad\qquad c_{2i} = c_o + \Delta_2 + \delta c_i \ (i = 1,\ldots,N)$$

$c_2 = c_o + \Delta_2$ denotes the new mean velocity and δc_i are the random changes. For a given frequency f, consider the change in the echo caused by going from c_1 to $c_2 = \{c_{2i}\}$. Thus write p_K at c_2 in terms of p_K at c_1:

$$p_K(c_2) = p_K(c_1) - \frac{\pi a^2}{\lambda^3} \sum_{i=1}^{N} \frac{\kappa_1 - \kappa_{2i}}{\kappa_o} I_i \tag{3}$$

Putting $\beta_i = \dfrac{\Delta_2 + \delta c_i}{c_o}$, $\quad \varepsilon = \dfrac{\Delta_1}{c_c}$, equation (3) becomes

$$p_K(c_2) = \frac{\pi a^2}{\lambda^3} \sum_{i=1}^{N} \left[\frac{\kappa_1}{\kappa_o} \frac{(1 + \varepsilon)^2}{(1 + \beta_i)^2} - 1 \right] I_i \tag{4}$$

$(1 + \beta_i)^{-2}$ has a pole at -1, however, $\beta_i = -1$ implies $c_{2i} = 0$, which is impossible. Nevertheless, for small negative values of β_i, this

factor can become very large, especially for c_2 similar to c_0.   If
c_2 c_0, the error is very small.

These theoretical considerations were confirmed by computer
calculations of regular and random hexagonal arrays for velocity
distributions about different means (see Fig. 3.).   The mean square
error (m.s.e.) was calculated w.r.t. the same hexagonal array of
constant velocity.   The error for random arrays was always larger than
for the respective regular arrays.   For the regular array with mean
velocity 2.68 and s.d. = 20%, the m.s.e. was always less than 4%,
while for the regular array with mean velocity 1.585 and s.d. = 10%,
the m.s.e. reaches 20%.

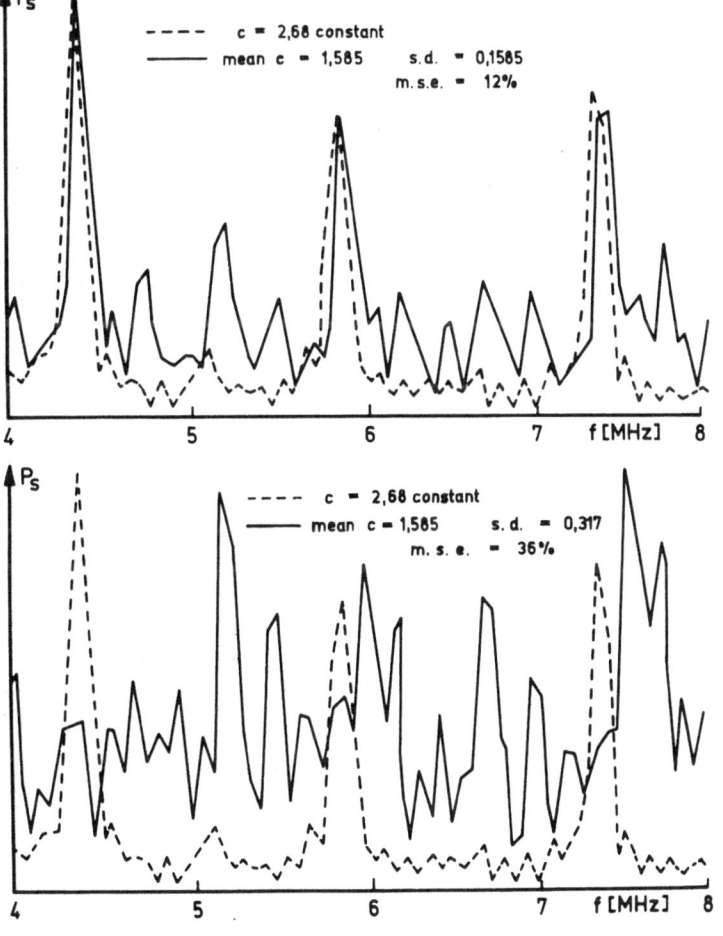

Fig. 3.   Backscattered pressure for random velocities.
(hexagonal arrays   0° regular)

SUMMARY AND DISCUSSION

In an attempt to characterize echoes from muscle tissue obtained from scanning by ultrasound, a model of the backscattered pressure as a function of frequency is applied to different scattering targets. Arrays of cylindrical scatterers were considered, and it was shown that important features occurring in the pressure spectra of regular arrays were preserved in the average of echoes from random arrays.

Simple data analysis was carried out. The autocorrelation techniques are generally less successsful for two-dimensional arrays than for one row only. However, they point towards analyzing echoes from planes rather than from individual scatterers. The cross-correlations proved to be a superior method of analysis to the auto-correlations. In particular, it seems promising to crosscorrelate spectra to be interpreted with those of known properties. From comparisons of these crosscorrelations with the respective auto-correlations of the known scattering targets, one could derive structural properties of the spectrum in question.

The effect of different velocities in the scatterers was also examined. The different velocities express different elastic properties of the tissue which could be caused by diseases. For a propagation velocity in the scatterers, which is not very different from that of the surrounding medium, the pressure spectrum becomes very sensitive even to small random changes in the velocity. There is hope that this method, applied to muscle tissue, will allow a differentiation between the velocity in diseased muscle and the average velocity of normal muscle.

REFERENCES

1. J. J. Faran, Jr., Sound scattering by solid cylinders and spheres, J. Acoust. Soc. Am. 23:405-418 (1951).
2. L. Fellingham-Joynt, A stoachastic approach to ultrasonic tissue characterization, Stanford University Thesis (June 1979).
3. J. C. Gore and S. Leeman, Ultrasonic backscattering from human tissue: a realistic model, Phys. Med. Biol. 22:317-326 (1977).
4. L. P. Hunter, P. P. K. Lee and R. C. Wang, Forward sound scat-tering by small nylon cylinders in water, J. Acoust. Soc. Am. 68 (1):314-319 (1980).
5. I. Koch and M. J. Eberle, A spherical wave model of ultrasonic backscattering from arrays of cylinders. To be published.
6. P. M. Morse and K. U. Ingard, "Theoretical Acoustics", McGraw Hill (1968).
7. D. Nicholas, An introduction to the theory of acoustic scattering by biological tissues, in: "Recent Advances in Ultrasound in Biomedicine 1", D. N. White, ed., Research Studies Press, (1977).

TISSUE CHARACTERIZATION OF NORMAL AND DYSTROPHIC MUSCLE USING

BROAD-BAND BACKSCATTERED R.F. DATA

E. B. Cady and J. E. Gardener

Department of Medical Physics and Bioengineering
University College Hospital, First Floor, Shropshire House
11-20 Capper Street, London WC1E 6JA, Great Britain

INTRODUCTION

There are many potential uses for the non-invasive "in vivo" characterization of muscle tissue. Dystrophic diseases produce large structural changes with a range of scale sizes comparable with fibres and fasciculi, introducing the possibility of quantitative monitoring by ultrasonic tissue characterization. The application of ultrasound to muscle disease has so far been limited and used mostly to determine approximate muscle volumes[1,2]. Some work has been done on the relationship of B-scan texture to the severity and type of muscular dystrophy[3] but no rigorous quantitative study has been attempted. The ultimate aim of the research is to provide a quantitative method for monitoring and diagnosing disease using modified conventional clinical equipment.

Muscle presents many difficulties for tissue characterization. The anisotropic nature of the fascicular architecture implies that tissue properties have to be measured as a function of probe/fasciculus inclination in order to ascertain whether any variations with angle are important. Values for the ultrasonic parameters of muscle can be found in the literature and many show an angle dependence[4]. The velocity of pulse propagation and the attenuation may be different along when compared with across the fibres[5].

For the technique to be of clinical use it is first necessary to characterize healthy muscle tissue and then to find the variances of parameters within the normal population and for various pathologies. Different muscles must be studied individually because they all have their own fascicular, vascular and connective tissue structures and scale sizes.

Great changes in the fascicular structure are produced in diseases such as the various muscular dystrophies. It is to be expected that the gross changes in structure caused by the replacement of fibres by fat and connective tissue will have a very marked effect on the ultrasonic characteristics of the muscle. Generally, a proportion of muscle fibres undergo necrosis, phagocytosis and eventual replacement by fat or connective tissue but each pathology has its own degenerative path. The structural changes are not uniform. Normal and regenerating tissue can be found alongside areas of dystrophied muscle.

THE SYSTEM

The following constraints apply to the technieques investigated:

(a) Data must be acquired by a single probe.

(b) Data must be collected easily and quickly.

(c) The techniques must be as system independent as possible.

(d) Additional equipment must be connected easily to the existing system.

(e) Probe dependent variations must have a minimal effect on the analysis techniques in order that comparable transducers can be easily constructed.

In order to obtain the fullest information on scattering structures in muscle tissue, it is necessary to:

(a) Use the largest possible signal bandwidth.

(b) Record the position and orientation of the interrogating transducer.

(c) Ensure that the sampled volume is located entirely within the muscle.

The system developed at U. C. H. is shown in Fig. 1. The basic scanner is a Nuclear Enterprises Diasonograph and gray-scale images are produced by a PEP 500 scan-converter. The front end of the system has been modified to include a Metrotek pulser and a variable gain pre-amplifier made by the G. E. C. Hirst Research Centre. The pre-amplifier is mounted close to the transducer and can provide a time programmable gain of up to 40 dB.

The transducers used for muscle studies have center frequencies of about 7 MHz, 50% bandwidths and diameters of 0.5 cm. Both

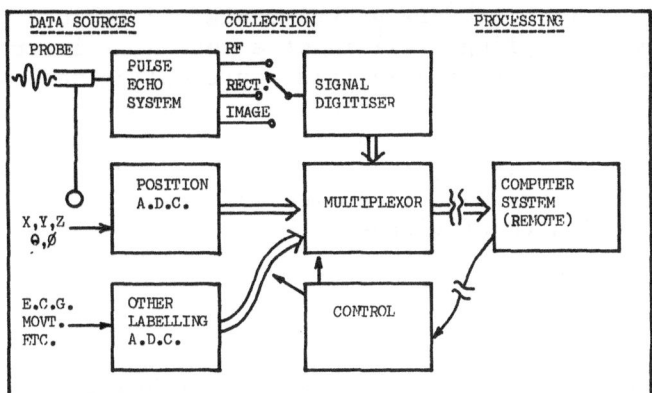

Fig. 1.

focussed and unfocussed versions have been used, the former having a
focal length of about 2 cm. Examination of a standard Graphite/
Gelatine phantom revealed no significant difference in visual texture
for any of the probes. Detailed numerical texture analysis (to be
described later) showed no difference between the transducers when
the experimental accuracy was considered.

Using a system bandwidth of approximately 12 MHz, the R. F.
output from the pre-amplifier is further amplified, filtered and
buffered before digitizing. The digitized signal is thus processed
entirely outside the Diasonograph imaging system. The digitizer is
a Biomation 8100 transient recorder which records 2048 8 bit samples
at a maximum rate of 100 MHz. The instrument operates under full
computer control and provides real time adjustment of sensitivity and
depth delay. Thus the system is capable of tracking a section of
muscle even if the depth changes and the attenuation due to overlying
tissue results in changes in signal level. The position at which
samples are recorded is set by computer monitoring of markers on the
image and on the A-mode display of the scanner.

In addition to the R. F. records up to 16 analogue signals from
the transducer position sensors are digitized and recorded to an
accuracy of 12 bits. Thus a complete reconstructed image can be
generated if desired, or alternatively, studies can be made of the
angular dependence of the back-scattered signal. Several of these
outputs are also available for recording control signals such as
cardiac phase or muscle position and tension. The computer system
comprises a PDP 11/45 mini-computer together with a PDP 11/10
machine as a front end buffer. The PDP 11/10 also sets up the
digitizer control commands, collects the data records sent from the
remote interface unit, tests for a "sampling" criterion and when
satisfied stores the data record on disk. The conditions for

acceptance of a data block are programmable and include probe motion
sensing, periodic sampling, fill in of a region of interest and manual
sampling requests. Operating in this way sampling rates of 100-200
records per second may be maintained. In order to ensure adequate
sampling of the R. F. waveform and taking into account the 12 MHz
system bandwidth, a sampling rate of 50 MHz has been used. In the
research described here data is collected in samples of 1024 points
corresponding to 1.4 cm of tissue.

DATA COLLECTION TECHNIQUE

     A suitable section of muscle has to be found before collecting
data. The muscle must be large enough to contain the gated length
of R. F. Regions showing large intrusions of connective tissue are
avoided. Using the image markers to ensure that the interrogated
volume is entirely within the muscle envelope, several (usually 16)
samples of data are collected at each of about 10 probe angles
covering a range including an inclination perpendicular to the
fasciculi. At every angle different samples are taken after shifting
the transducer a few millimeters across the muscle. Between each
set of samples the probe has its inclination altered by a few degrees
and is locked in position. It is vital that the patient is kept as
still as possible throughout this process so as not to disturb the
probe/muscle geometry.

ANALYSIS TECHNIQUE

     A 1-Dimensional texture analysis method[6] has been used in which
it is hypothesized that the important features in a given texture
are the relative amplitudes of adjacent "bright" and "dark" areas.
In this method the data are smoothed by a "backlash" algorithm
which removes adjacent maxima and minima when the difference in
amplitude is less than a certain threshold. The basic process is
described adequately in the reference given. The total number of
maxima and minima remaining is determined and the threshold is
increased. Repeated application of the algorithm gives a function
describing the variation of the number of extrema with increasing
threshold.

     A preliminary investigation of the texture parameters and their
variances indicated that the most sensitive results were obtained
using R. F. rather than demodulated data. This must be due to the
fact that the R. F. signal has phase information and the bandwidth
is larger. It was also decided that some adaptations to the process
described in (6) would be necessary if it were to utilize fully the
information present in the R. F. data. Firstly a correction was
made for changes in echo amplitude caused by attenuation within the
tissue. This produced an echo train stationary with respect to

amplitude. With the data corrected for attenuation it was no longer
necessary to use logarithmic amplitude as described in (6). This
was advantageous because the logarithmic processing biases the
technique towards low amplitude data which, in the R. F. case, contain
minimal textural information. The data were normalized so that the
average R. F. amplitude was 100 arbitrary units and thresholds were
set at 10, 20, 30 ... on the same scale. By taking ratios of the
number of extrema at one threshold to the number at the next, a
texture feature is obtained that is independent of the length of the
sampled volme. These ratios were used in all the analyses so that
direct comparison could be made with results obtained using shorter
or longer time gates.

RESULTS

(a)   Graphite/Gelatine Phantom

     The phantom used during the research consisted of a Graphite/
Gelatine material[7] and was very useful in the texture analysis
for the comparison of transducers and monitoring long term variations
in a particular probe. Fig. 2. shows results for 5 different probes.

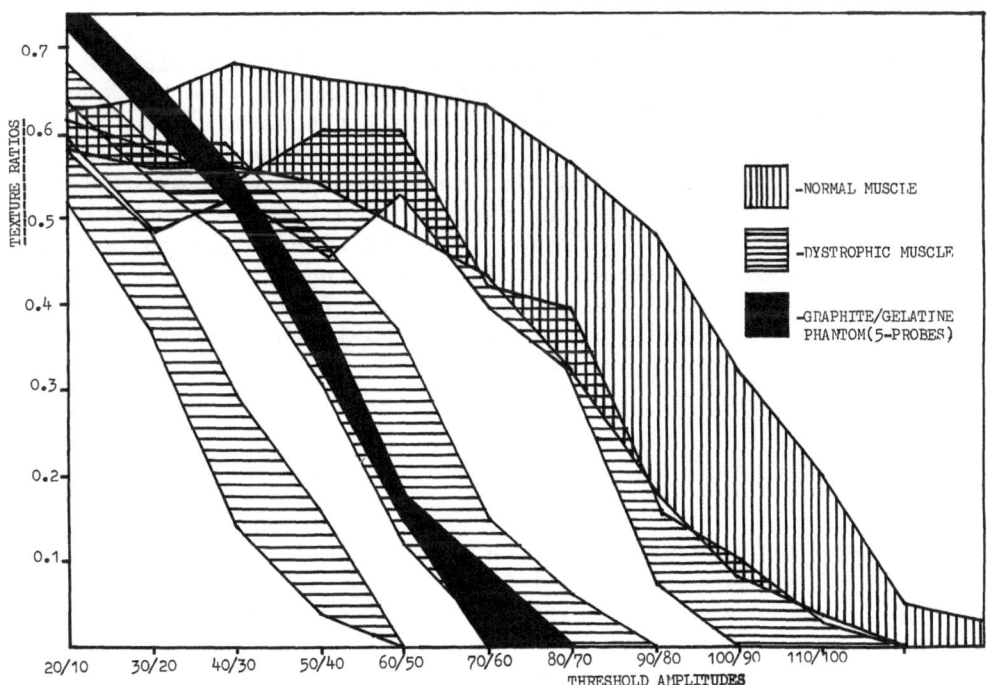

Fig. 2.   Texture ratios for normal and dystrophic muscle tissue and
          for 5 different transducers+Graphite/Gelatine phantom.

(b) In "vivo"

In "vivo" data have been acquired from normal and pathological
muscles. The Tibialis Anterior and Vastus Intermedius have been
investigated in detail because of their size, accessibility and
uniform fascicular architecture. Preliminary investigations of other
muscles (e.g. Vastus Lateralis, Rectus Femoris, Adductor Magnus,
Biceps Brachii and Erector Spinalis) have been made in order to
assess their suitability for examination.

Several immediate observations can be made concerning the
appearance of normal and pathological tissue on B-scans. Most
obvious is the textural difference in the muscle parenchyma. In
images of normal muscle some angle dependent phenomena are seen.
The bone echo is strong and muscle envelopes are clearly seen if
the probe is correctly inclined during scanning. Images of the
normal parenchyma range from conspicuous striations or solitary
echoes to almost completely anechoic. In the case of dystrophic
tissue[3] attenuation seems to be higher, muscle envelopes are
difficult to see and in advanced cases the normally strong bone echo
is absent (in spite of the thinness of the wasted limb). Figs. 3
and 4 show B-scans of a normal and a dystrophic thigh. The muscle
textures in the images are clearly different.

Useful results were obtained from the quantitative texture
analysis (Fig. 2.). No significant systematic angle dependence was
found over the range used although the back-scattered amplitude
varies considerably. Variances for some thresholds were between
15 and 25% of the mean value. Data from all the normal muscles
were comparable and there was little variation between individuals.
These results can be contrasted with data from patients with advanced
forms of muscular dystrophy. The dystrophic data show a much larger
range of textures than the normals. This is to be expected because
the patients examined were all at different stages in the advancement
of their disease and also the severity varies from muscle to muscle.
An indicator of the usefulness of the method is the fact that the
degree of textural change is proportional to the stage of advancement
of the disease.

CONCLUSIONS

The consistent results obtained show that is is possible to
adapt existing clinical equipment to enable the quantitative
assessment of back-scattered signals. The very significant
difference between normal and pathological results indicates that
the method has a potential for monitoring and staging dystrophic
disease in individual muscles.

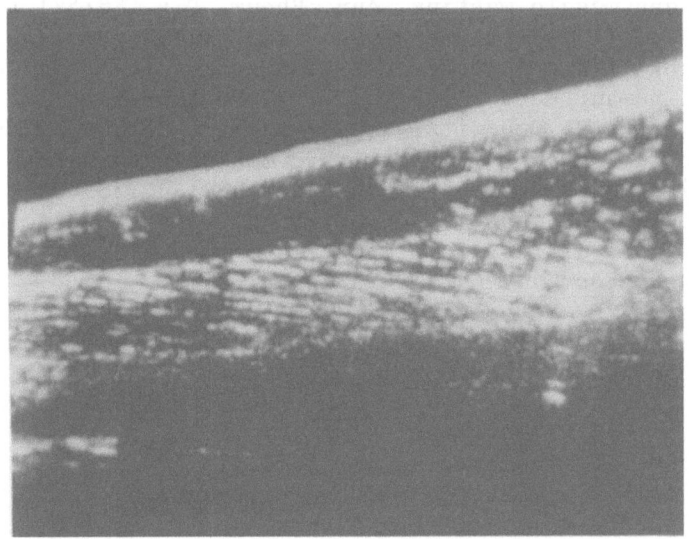

Fig. 3. Normal muscle. Anterior sagittal view of Vastus Intermedius
and Rectus Femoris

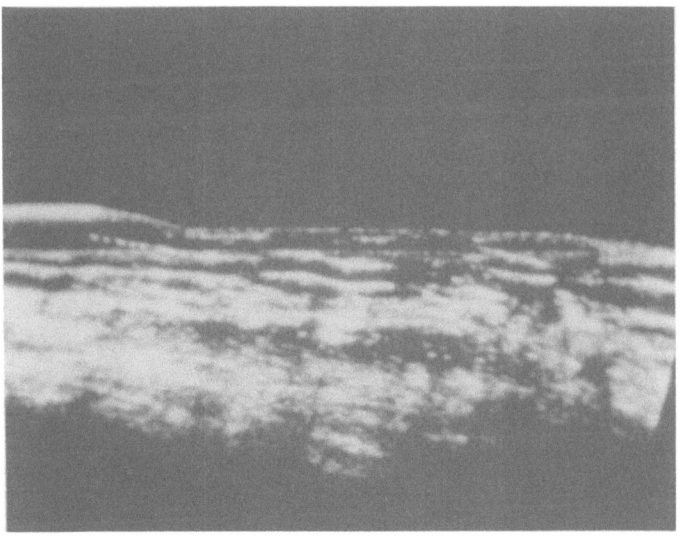

Fig. 4. Dystrophic muscle. Similar view to Fig. 3.

REFERENCES

1. A. Young, I. Hughes, P. Russell, and M. J. Parker, Measurement of
   Quadriceps muscle wasting, Ann. Rheum. Dis. 38:571 (1979).
2. B. Dons, K. Bollerup, F. Bonde-Petersen, and S. Hancke, The effect
   of weight lifting exercise related to muscle cross sectional
   area in human, Eur. Jl. Physiol. 40:95 (1979).
3. J. Z. Heckmatt, V. Dubowitz, and S. Leeman, Detection of
   pathological change in dystrophic muscle with B-scan ultrasound imaging, The Lancet, 28 June 1980, p.1389.
4. S. A. Goss, R. L. Johnston, and F. Dunn, Comprehensive compilation
   of empirical ultrasonic properties of mammalian tissues,
   J. Acoust. Soc. Am. 64(2):423 (1978).
5. D. K. Nassiri, D. Nicholas, and C. R. Hill, Attenuation of
   ultrasound in skeletal muscle, Ultrasonics :280 (1979).
6. O. R. Mitchell, C. R. Myers, and W. Boyne, A max. min. measure
   for image texture analysis, IEEE Trans. Computers C26:408
   (1977).
7. E. L. Masden, J. A. Zagzebski, R. A. Banjavic, and R. E. Jutila,
   Tissue mimicking materials for ultrasound phantoms, Med. Phys.
   5:391 (1978).

SOME RESULTS ON ULTRASONIC TISSUE CHARACTERIZATION*

J. M. Thijssen, A. L. Bayer and M. Cloostermans

Biophysics Laboratory of the Department of Ophthalmology
University of Nijmegen,
6500 HB Nijmegen, The Netherlands

INTRODUCTION

In this paper various approaches developed during the last few years are presented. The data given have been published previously in some form. The subjects discussed are: statistical analysis of A-mode video echograms[1,2], including a few clinical results; methods of characterization of membranes, including a few in vivo data[3,4]; and finally, methods of characterization of tissues by analysis of backscattered ultrasound[5,6].

The A-mode video analysis has been applied in clinical routine for some time and its feasibility and significance have already been shown by the authors[7]. The acoustic characterization of membranes has been developed for ophthalmological applications, i.e. the differentiation of intraocular membranes.

Another application may be impediography, which may yield a valuable tissue parameter. Ultrasonic tissue characterization is also the purpose of the spectral analysis of backscattered RF echograms. This kind of analysis yields the so-called tissue transfer function[8,9], which results in a one parameter description of the dispersion in the attenuation coefficient. For further reference other publications [10,11] have been mentioned.

METHODS

The scheme showing the equipment used is depicted in Fig. 1.

─────────────
*This work has been supported by The Health Organization -- THO.

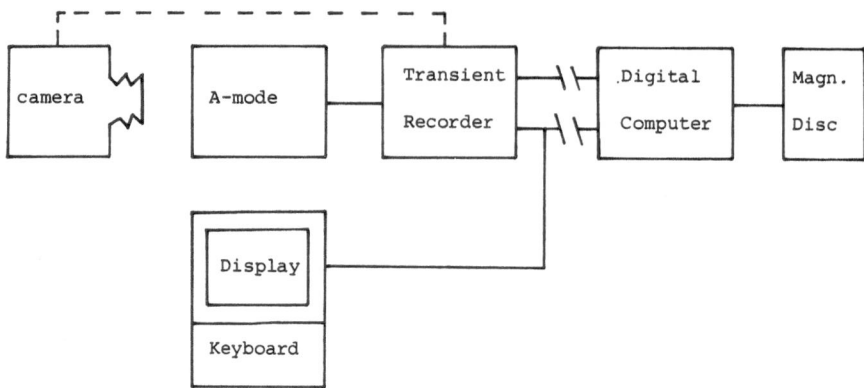

Fig. 1. Data acquisition is initiated either by taking a photograph
         of the A-mode image, or by software control. The data are
         sampled, digitized and stored in an appropriate rate by a
         transient recorder. Data are then transferred to disk by
         a digital computer. Communication with the computer is
         possible from the examination room (after Thijssen et al.[1])

The data acquisition is triggered by taking a photograph of the
A-mode screen (in case of video analysis), or alternatively pressing
a switch on the transient recorder (Biomation 8100). The acquisition
of video signals proceeds as follows: after the first echogram is
digitized (10 MHz 512 samples) the computer (PDP 11/34) reads it into
the memory and commands a new acquisition cycle. The transient
recorder is then triggered by the next coming transmission pulse of
the A-mode equipment (Kretztechnik 7200 MA) and the whole cycle is
repeated until 24 echograms are stored. The time it takes for
completing the data acquisition is 3 seconds. During this time the
manually applied ultrasound transducer may move slightly due to
involuntary movements of the operator and the patient, and so does
the sound beam with respect to the pathology. The quality of the
stored echograms is examined by a so-called DOT-display of the
maxima (i.e. individual ehco peaks) of the successively stored echograms (Fig. 2.).

    The radiofrequency echograms are obtained by using a homemade
transmitter-receiver and a special broadband transducer ($\emptyset$ = 17 mm,
focus 60 mm) with a 40 mm water stand-off. The transient recorder
is now employed in a 50 MHz sampling rate and a maximum of 25
echograms (512 samples) can be stored then in 0.6 seconds. This high
rate is required now, because it is necessary to average the RF echograms in order to improve the signal to noise ratio. The noise is
partly of electronic nature (receiver) and partly caused by the poor
behavior of the transient recorder at the 50 MHz sampling rate
(multiplicative digitization noise, c.f. Bayer and Thijssen[4]). The

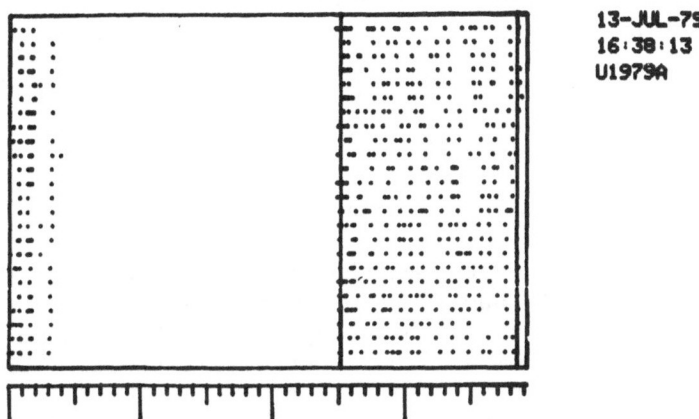

Fig. 2. Dot display of 24 echographic sweeps (A-mode echograms)
showing the echopeaks like dots. Horizontal rows correspond
to successive sweeps.

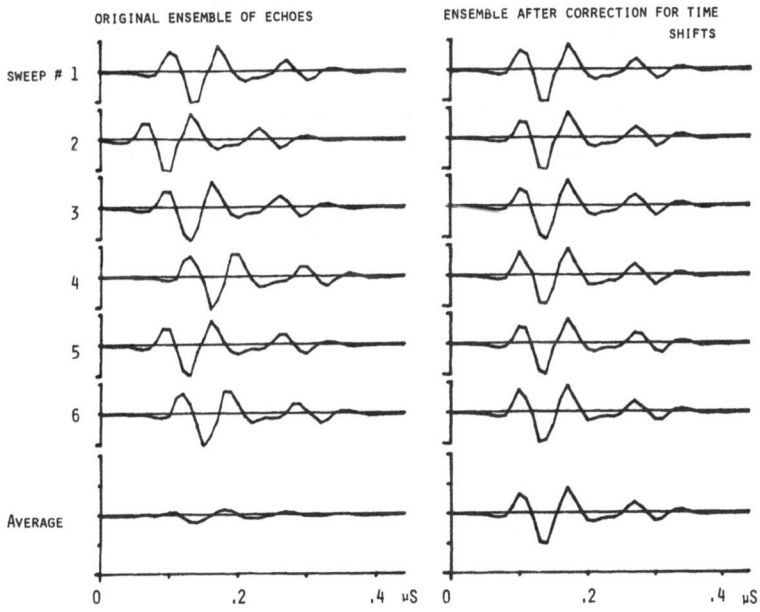

Fig. 3. Left: Original RF echograms, note the misalignment caused
by electronic jitter, and hand movements.
Right: Same echograms after alignment by a computer program
(after Bayer and Thijssen[3].

averaging procedure we have developed includes phase correction and
DC drifting, the resulting improvement by the alignment can be
decided from Fig. 3.

RESULTS

Tissue Characterization from A-Mode Video Echograms

        An example of the output of the program for statistical analysis
is shown in Fig. 4. It should be mentioned first that the data used
for the anlysis comprise all the echopeaks within a selected region
(region of interest) from all the 24 echograms stored. The left-hand
pictures in Fig. 4. display a single, and the average echogram,
respectively. The expanded view of the region of interest is shown
in the upper middle picture. The oblique line drawn in this picture
(as well as in the lower left one) displays the regression line
through the peaks in the region of interest. Since the magnitude
of the echoes is not only determined by the reflectivity and the
attenuation of the tissues but also by the gain compression by the
video amplifier, we have to correct the data prior to analysis. This
correction is possible by using a special electronic device (electronic tissue model[12]) and after reading this gain compression
curve into the computer.

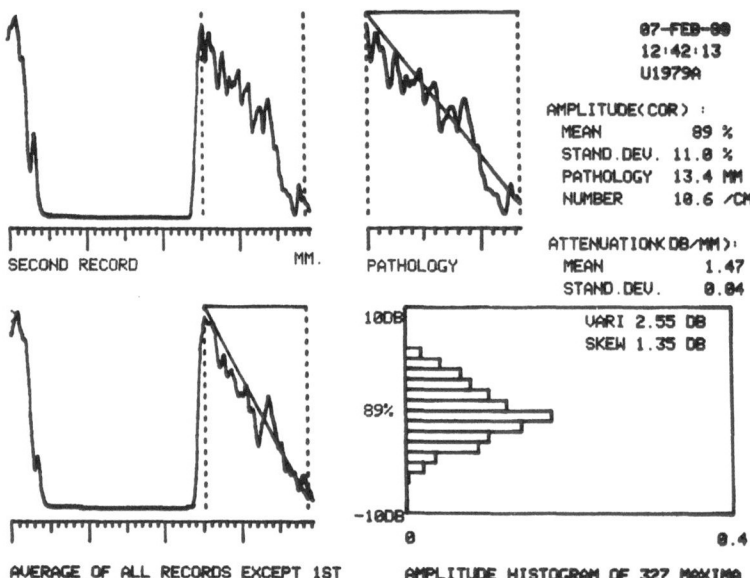

Fig. 4. Output of statistical analysis of video echograms. Region
         of interest (between dotted lines): normal orbital fat
         (after Thijssen et al.[1]).

The data given in the top right of Fig. 4. gives some
statistical measures like mean reflectivity (relative to maximum
display magnitude and by using a standard sensitivity setting of
the equipment) and regression. The regression is to be considered
as a first estimate of the attenuation, because the ultrasonic
equipment has a relatively narrow bandwidth. The histogram (bottom
right) in Fig. 4. has been rotated 90° so that the amplitudes are
at the ordinate. It is primarily meant to investigate whether the
texture of the echogram is uniquely represented in this histogram.
Our results[7] on intra-ocular tumors revealed a regression of
0.8 dB/mm which is about one half of the value found for orbital
fat, and an amplitude level of 33%, with a standard deviation of
2 dB with respect to the regression line. The number of echoes
detected by the computer program is on average 7.5 per cm, while
for the orbital fat 10.5 peaks per cm are found. The differentiation
of focal and diffuse orbital lesions especially may become an
important application of this kind of statistical analysis.

Membrane Characterization from RF Echograms

We have chosen the inverse filtering technique as a means of
deconvolving the echograms and by this revealing the exact time,
phase and amplitude of the interface echoes. The technique is
schematically outlined in Fig. 5.

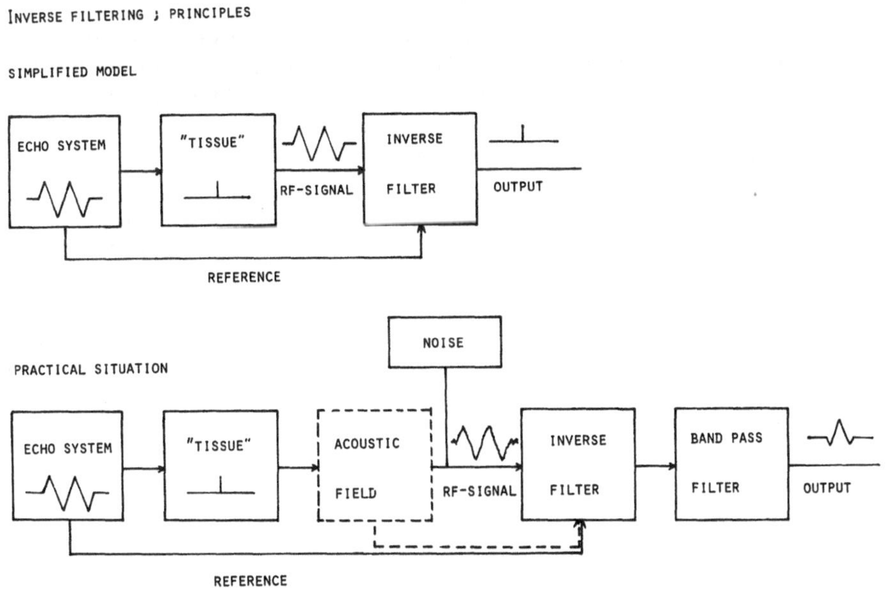

Fig. 5. Upper part: Scheme of echo formation and deconvolution by
                     inverse filtering.
         Lower part: Practical situation involving noise and sound
                     field effects (after Bayer and Thijssen[3]).

The basic assumption is that an echo may be considered as the result of a convolution of a point event (δ-function) with a fixed waveform (reference echo) produced by the echographic equipment. This assumption implies that no frequency dependent interaction of the ultrasound with biological tissues takes place. In practice both frequency dependent attenuation and reflection occur and additionally the received signal is disturbed by noise. This implies that the echograms have to be improved by, for instance, averaging and band filtering algorithms. This all results in a considerable decrease in the exactness in the estimation of the acoustic parameters we are interested in. The results we are obtaining after applying the various methods of improvement are encouraging[3,4]. The broadening of the bandwidth and the resulting enhancement of the resolution in the time domain is of the order of a factor of two. The most promising technique appears to be a combination of a Wiener inverse filter and a one sided Hanning filter[4].

The data from an in vitro measurement of a polyethylene foil and using a Hanning inverse filter are shown in Fig. 6. The same type of filter was applied to the data in the right hand part of Fig. 6., which were measured in vivo in a case of retinal detachment.

Spectral Analysis of Tissue Echograms

We have performed in vitro measurements in order to investigate the limitations and accuracy limits of the technique that has been outlined by Kuc and Schwartz[9]. The first subject concerned the influence of the sound field. It could be demonstrated that for a focused transducer the high frequency part of the spectrum is suppressed before and after the focus[5]. This effect could be described analytically[6], so it is possible to correct for it if the correction is estimated for the transducer used. The procedure in the in vitro experiments comprises not only averaging in the time domain of 200 sweeps, but also a kind of spatial averaging after repeating the measurement at 35 different positions with respect to the tissue sample. The echograms are segmented by applying a Hanning time window of 3 microseconds half width. The power spectra of the small pieces of the echograms are then calculated per position and the average is taken over the 35 positions (Fig. 7.).

Next the power spectra of the first one third of the echogram are divided by those of the last third. The resulting relative spectra are, therefore, obtained from identically separated positions in depth and may be averaged. The resulting data are displayed in Fig. 8. (cf. Fig. 7.).

The attenuation slope for liver tissue is (1.0 $\pm$ 0.1) dB/cm/MHz. The standard deviation of 0.1 dB/cm/MHz is caused by the spatial distribution of the scatterers in the tissue. Further investigations

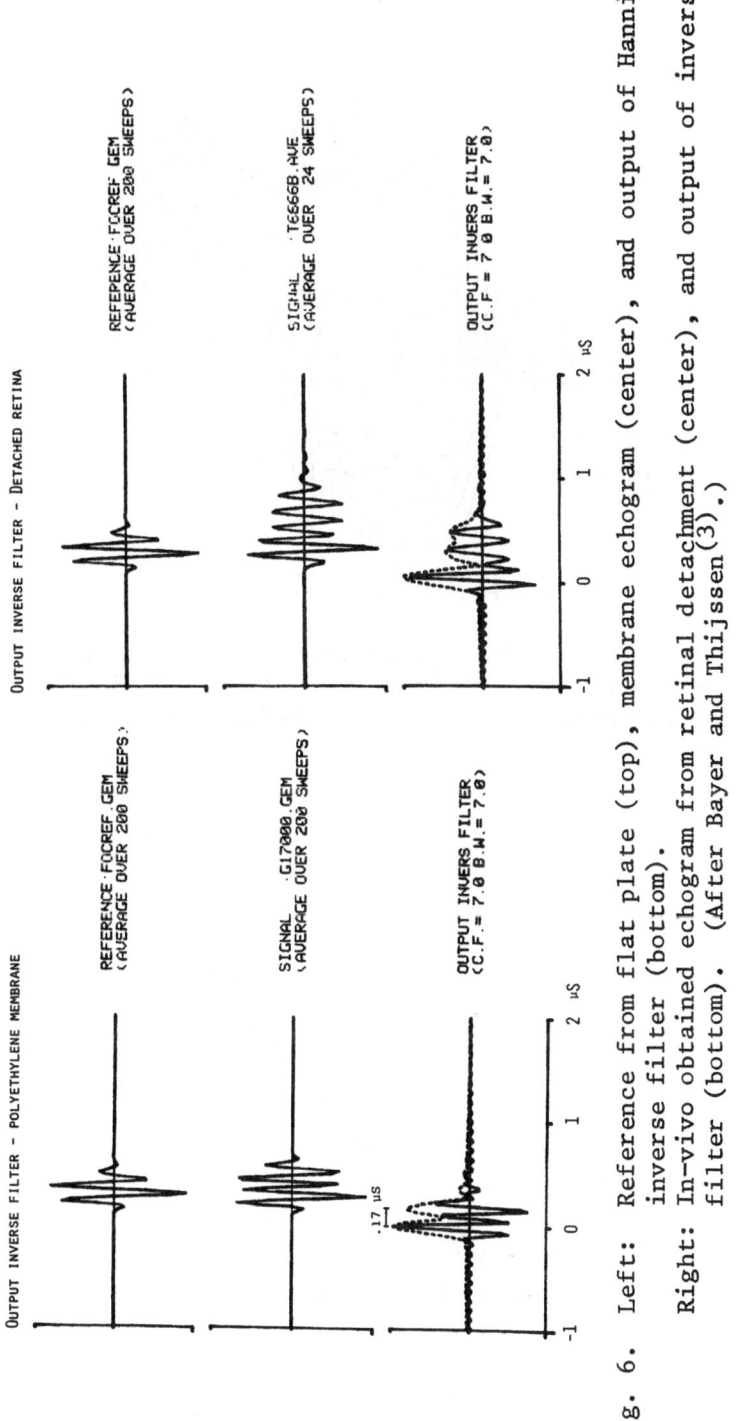

Fig. 6. Left: Reference from flat plate (top), membrane echogram (center), and output of Hanning inverse filter (bottom).

Right: In-vivo obtained echogram from retinal detachment (center), and output of inverse filter (bottom). (After Bayer and Thijssen[3].)

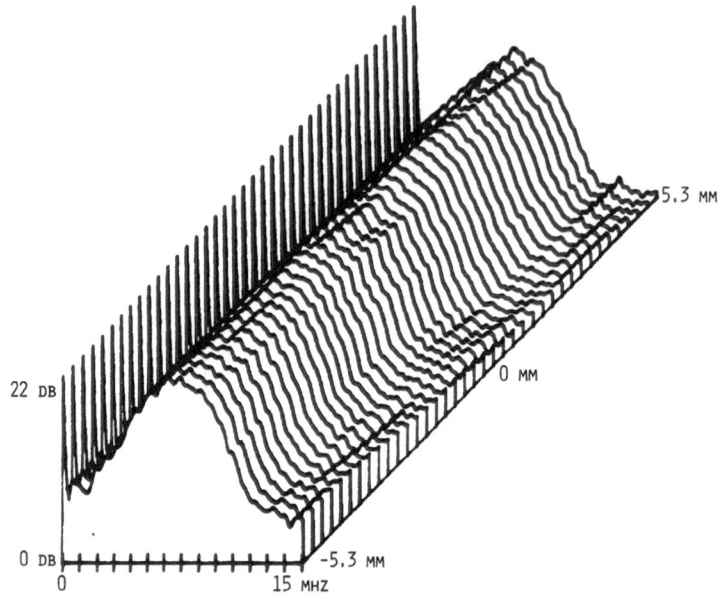

Fig. 7.   In vitro obtained power spectra as a function of depth in
          the liver tissue. The gradual suppression of higher
          frequencies is to be noted (after Thijssen et al.[5]).

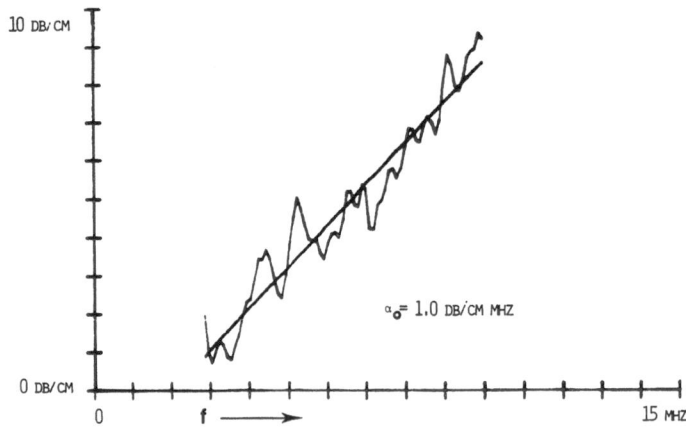

Fig. 8.   Attenuation slope of liver tissue from Fig. 7. (after
          Thijssen et al.[5].)

are needed to achieve a technique that can be used in in vivo examinations while the accuracy is maintained at the level we attained. It is, however, without any doubt, that a very important step towards ultrasonic tissue differentiation is made and that acoustospectrography may become a highly appreciated diagnostic tool.

REFERENCES

1. J. M. Thijssen, A. L. Bayer, and M. Cloostermans, Computer assisted echography: statistical analysis of A-mode video echograms obtained by tissue sampling, Med. Biol. Engng. & Comp. (in press).
2. J. M. Thijssen, R. Kruizinga, H. van Dooren, and A. M. Verbeek, Computer assisted echographic analysis, in: "Diagnostica Ultrasonic in Ophthalmologica", H. Gernet, ed., Remy Verl., Münster (1979), p.12-14.
3. A. L. Bayer and J. M. Thijssen, Characterization of intraocular membranes by means of inverse filtering, in: "Ultrasonography in Ophthalmology 8", Doc. Ophthal. Proc. Series, Vol. 29, J. M. Thijssen and A. M. Verbeek, eds., Junk, Den Haag (in press).
4. A. L. Bayer and J. M. Thijssen, Ultrasonic characterization of tissue interfaces by inverse filtering procedures, (in preparation).
5. J. M. Thijssen, M. Cloostermans, and A. L. Bayer, Measurement of ultrasonic attenuation in tissue from backscattered reflections, in: "Ultrasonography in Ophthalmology 8", Doc. Ophthal. Proc. Series, Vol. 29, J. M. Thijssen and A. M. Verbeek, eds., Junk, Den Haag (in press).
6. M. Cloostermans and J. M. Thijssen, Estimation of ultrasound attenuation slope from backscattering: in vitro assessment of field effects and of accuracy limits, (in preparation).
7. J. M. Thijssen and A. M. Verbeek, Computer analysis of A-mode echograms from choroidal melanoma, in: "Ultrasonography in Ophthalmology 8", Doc. Ophthal. Proc. Series, Vol. 29, J. M. Thijssen and A. M. Verbeek, eds., Junk, Den Haag (in press).
8. A. C. Kac and K. A. Dines, Signal processing of pulsed ultrasound, IEEE Transact. Biomed. Engng. 4:321 (1978).
9. R. Kac and M. Schwartz, Estimating the acoustic attenuation coefficient slope for liver from reflected ultrasound signals, IEEE Transaction SU 26:363 (1979).
10. J. M. Thijssen, ed., "Ultrasonic Tissue Characterization", Stafleu, Alphen a/d Rijn (1980).
11. J. M. Thijssen and A. M. Verbeek, eds., "Ultrasonography in Ophthalmology 8", Doc. Ophthal. Proc. Series, Vol. 29, Junk, Den Haag (in press).
12. S. J. H. Kervel and J. M. Thijssen, A device for the display and adjustment of the non-linear gain curve of ultrasonic A-mode equipment, Ultrasonics 19:40-42 (1981).

TISSUE CHARACTERIZATION BY ULTRASONIC PULSE SPECTROSCOPY

K. P. Richter, H. Heynemann, and R. Millner

Institute of Applied Biophysics and Department of
Urology, Martin-Luther-University, DDR 4014 Halle
Str. d. DSF 81

INTRODUCTION

The acoustic properties of biological tissues showed a
characteristic dependence on their specific structure. Ultrasonic
diagnosis in A- and B-mode techniques used the information from
reflected and backscattered signals of pulsed ultrasonic waves. But
more comprehensive signal processing allowed us to get more accurate
information concerning tissue structures. These new attempts use
techniques, e.g. impedography, time of flight tomography, computerized
ultrasonic tomography, and spectrum analysis[1,2,3,4].

In this way the frequency dependent ultrasonic attenuation,
backscattering and velocity measurements become important in
distinguishing between normal and pathological tissues[5]. Many
attempts were made to utilize these specific properties and new
methods in signal processing leading to the current spectrum analysis
of echoes and echo groups[6]. In comparison with the histological
state we tried to find out a correlation between the clinical
statement and the frequency dependent ultrasonic attenuation[7].

MATERIALS AND METHODS

In vitro measurements of fixed tissues were performed in degassed water. A series of normal and pathological human testes were
studied. The specimens were cut in parallel slices. Ten measurements
on each preparation and different specimens with the same pathological
state provided a statistical mean for the measured data. The
attenuation measurements were carried out with an A-scope device. A
broadband ultrasonic transducer with a center frequency of 6 MHz

95

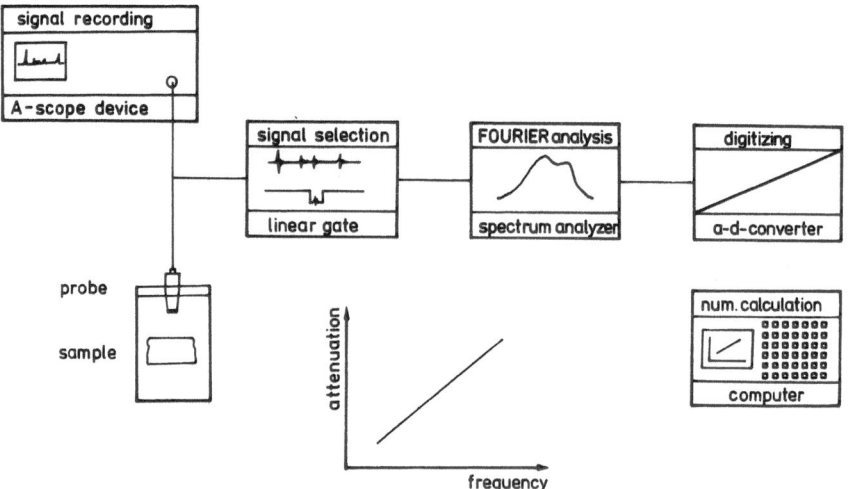

Fig. 1. Block diagram of the electronic device

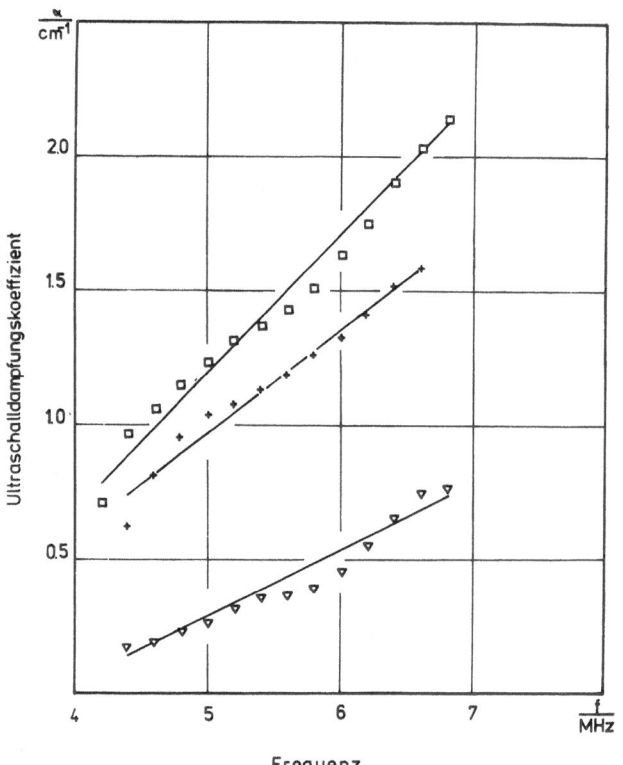

Fig. 2. Ultrasonic attenuation versus frequency
         tumor   + chronic inflammation   ∇ normal testis

served for a wide frequency range. We used a modified A-scope
device, as shown in Fig. 1., followed by a linear gate and an
electronic spectrum analyzer. From the digitized spectra the
computation of attenuation was performed by a calculator. Measurements in transmission and pulse-echo-technique were carried out.

RESULTS AND DISCUSSION

    With these methods we observed a different ultrasonic
attenuation between normal, neoplastic, and chronically inflamed
tissues. Characteristic results of the frequency dependent ultrasonic attenuation are represented in Figs. 2. and 3. Thereby a
remarkable difference between the very low attenuation of the normal
and the high attenuation of the pathological specimen is seen. The
neoplastic data differ also from the chronically inflamed tissues.
A differentiation between different tumor groups being the subject
of our current investigations has not yet been completed.

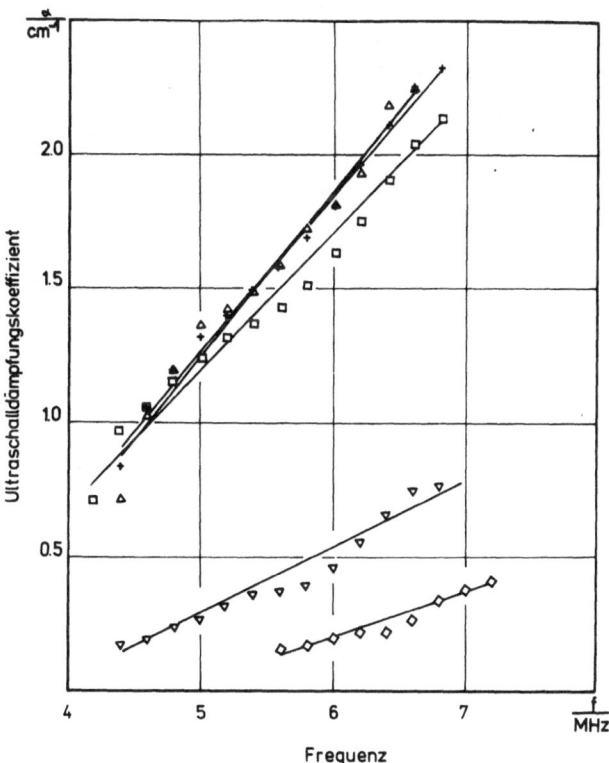

Fig. 3. Ultrasonic attenuation versus frequency
         Δ + tumor   ∇ normal testis

CONCLUSION

The ultrasonic pulse spectroscopy allowed a differentiation between normal and pathological tissues of testes in vitro. We found remarkable changes between normal tissue and chronically inflamed or neoplastic tissues. The preliminary investigations prompt us to carry out a more in depth examination and transferance of this technique to in vivo conditions.

REFERENCES

1. J. P. Jones, Ultrasonic impediography and its application to tissue characterization, in: "Recent Advances in Ultrasound in Biomedicine, Vol. 1", D. N. White, ed., Research Studies Press, Forest Grove, Oregon (1977), p.131-155.
2. G. H. Glover and J. C. Sharp, Reconstruction of ultrasound propagation speed distributions in soft tissue: time of flight tomography, IEEE Trans. Son. Ultrason. SU-24/4:229-234 (1977).
3. H. Schomberg, Nonlinear image reconstruction from projections of ultrasonic travel times and electric current densities, in: "Lecture Notes in Medical Information", G. T. Herman and F. Natterer, eds., Springer, New York (1980), p.124-147.
4. J. C. Boboux, F. Lakestani, P. Fleischmann, M. Perdix, C. Guillaud and R. Groutte, An ultrasonic spectroscopy device, application to tissue differentiation, in: "Excerpta Medica International Congress Series No. 363: Proceedings of the Second European Congress on Ultrasonics in Medicine, Munich, 12-16 May 1975", E. Kazner, H. R. Müller and M. de Vlieger, eds., Excerpta Medica, Amsterdam (1975), p.108-114.
5. P. N. T. Wells, Absorption and dispersion of ultrasound in biological tissue, Ultrasound in Med. Biol. 1:369 (1975).
6. R. C. Chivers, C. R. Hill and D. Nicholas, Frequency dependence of ultrasonic backscattering cross-sections, in: "Excerpta Medica International Congress Series No. 309: Proceedings of the Second World Congress on Ultrasonics in Medicine, Rotterdam, 4-8 June 1973", M. de Vlieger, D. N. White and V. R. McCready, eds., Excerpta Medica, Amsterdam (1973), p.300-303.
7. H. Heynemann and K. P. Richter, Neue Möglichkeiten der Hodentumordiagnostik mittels Ultraschallspektroskopie, in: "Proc. 15. Urologenkongress der DDR", (1980), p.256.

STUDY OF ULTRASONIC TOPOGRAPHY OF THE KIDNEY

A.P. Sarvazyan and V.A. Klemin

Institute of Biological Physics
Academy of Sciences of the USSR
Pushchino, Moscow Region, 142292, USSR

The increasing interest in the investigation of the acoustic characteristics of biological tissues which has occurred in the past decade is caused by the progress made in ultrasonic imaging in medical diagnostics. The possibility of obtaining ultrasonic images of biological substances is based on the acoustic heterogeneity of these structures. That is why the investigation of the acoustic topography of tissue, i.e. the spatial distribution of velocities and attenuation coefficients of ultrasonic waves and the changes in the acoustic topography during functional and parhological processes is of special importance.

The conventional methods of ultrasonic attenuation and velocity measurements in soft tissues require large volumes of material and are not able to provide data on the local ultrasonic characteristics of tissue necessary to study its acoustic topography. The spatial resolution of the measuring method must be of the order of millimeters, being comparable to the resolution of medical imaging devices. The second condition is the need for high sensitivity of the method in order to reveal small local differences in acoustic properties of tissues.

An apparatus which can satisfy both of these conditions has recently been developed by one of the authors[1]. This apparatus is based on the fixed path interferometric method. The velocity of ultrasound in the tissue, which is placed between two protruding ends of a fork shaped acoustic resonator, is determined by the frequency of the given resonance and the absorption is evaluated from the quality factor of the resonator. The volume of tissue needed for the measurement is equal to 3.5 mm x 3.5 mm x 1.2 mm. The velocity

can be measured with a precision of 0.03% and the attenuation measured
to about 5%. The measurements are performed at an operating frequency
of 8.8 MHz and a temperature of between 22–23°C.

The temperature of the tissue in the resonator cell was measured
by a thermocouple with a precision of ± 0.1°C. Dog kidneys were
investigated. Measurements were carried out on the freshly excised
kidneys and lasted about 5 hours. The fork shaped resonator allowed
for in-situ measurements by placing the measuring ends of the
resonator into small parallel cuts in the plane of the chosen kidney
cross section. The density of small pieces of tissue (± 0.1 cm^3),
taken from different parts of the kidney section under investigation,
were measured in parallel with the acoustic measurements. The density
of the tissues was estimated from the density of aqueous $CuSO_4$
solutions in which the sample was in a state of neutral equilibrium.
The acoustic impedances of the tissue samples were calculated from
the density data and the measured ultrasonic velocity.

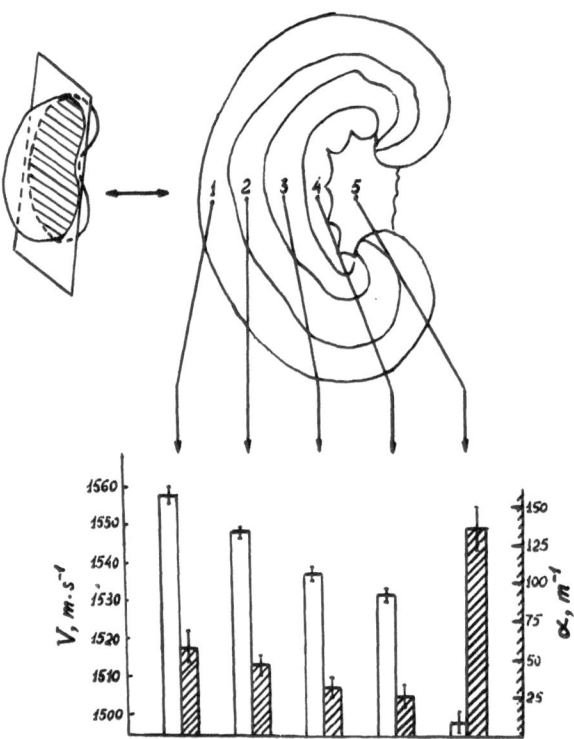

Fig. 1. Ultrasound velocity and attentuation coefficient in the
         five acoustically distinct regions of the longitudinal
         cross section of a dog kidney.

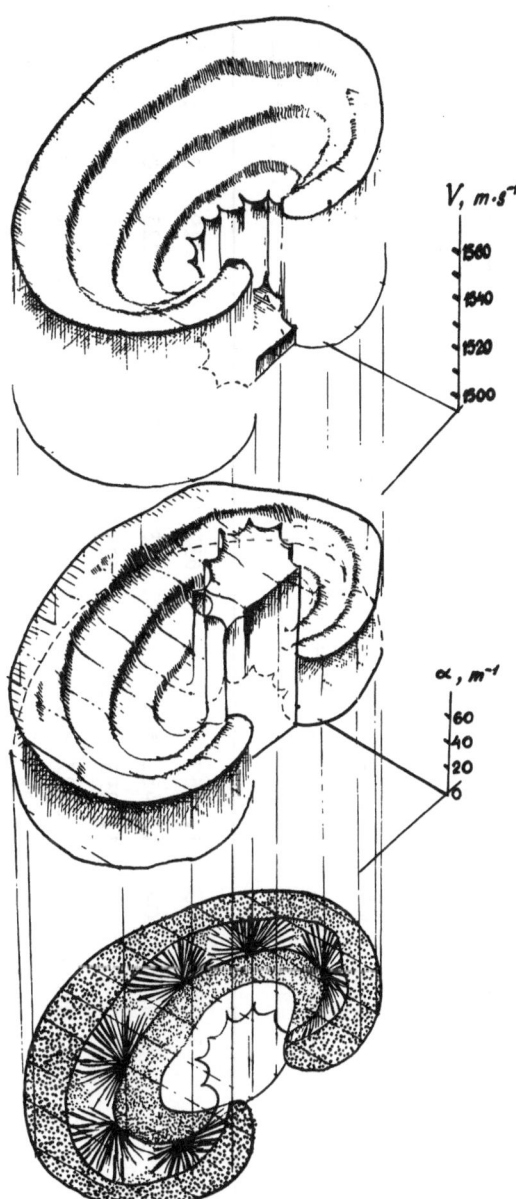

Fig. 2. Topographic sketch of ultrasound velocity and attenuation
         coefficient distribution in the longitudinal cross section
         of a dog kidney.

Table 1. Local acoustic characteristics of different sites of longitudinal cross sections of kidneys.

Number of kidney	Number of region	Number of site	Density g.cm^{-3}	Velocity V cm.s^{-1} x 10^{-5}	Acoustic Impedance I g.cm^{-2}.s^{-2} x 10^{-5}	Adiabatic compressibility, β cm^2.dyne^{-1} x 10^{11}	Attenuation coefficient α cm^{-1}
1	1	19	1.060±0.003	1.54860±0.0019	1.6415±0.0066	3.933±0.020	0.52±0.07
	2	17	1.056±0.004	1.53940±0.0021	1.6256±0.0084	3.996±0.019	0.42±0.06
	3	16	1.052±0.002	1.53660±0.0006	1.6165±0.0037	4.026±0.011	0.35±0.03
	4	10	1.048±0.002	1.5270±0.0004	1.600 ±0.0037	4.092±0.011	0.24±0.03
	5	5		1.487 ±0.002			1.25±0.15
2	1	16	1.062±0.003	1.5562 ±0.0016	1.632 ±0.0064	3.936±0.019	0.54±0.06
	2	16	1.058±0.004	1.5481 ±0.002	1.638 ±0.0083	3.944±0.025	0.47±0.06
	3	13	1.052±0.002	1.5395 ±0.0011	1.619 ±0.0042	4.011±0.013	0.34±0.04
	4	9	1.049±0.002	1.5327 ±0.0006	1.608 ±0.0038	4.058±0.011	0.30±0.03
	5	4		1.499 ±0.0025			1.23±0.12
3	1	18	1.060±0.003	1.5524 ±0.002	1.646 ±0.0068	3.915±0.021	0.56±0.07
	2	16	1.055±0.003	1.5464 ±0.0024	1.631 ±0.0072	3.964±0.023	0.44±0.07
	3	16	1.049±0.003	1.5369 ±0.0015	1.612 ±0.0062	4.036±0.019	0.36±0.05
	4	8	1.049±0.002	1.5307 ±0.001	1.606 ±0.0041	4.068±0.013	0.27±0.02
	5	4		1.490 ±0.002			1.30±0.2

Table 2. Relative values of the local acoustic characteristics of kidneys

Number of region	Number of Kidney	Number of sites	Values of the acoustic characteristics of different kidney regions related to those of the first region		
			V_i/V_1	I_i/I_1	α_i/α_1
2	1	17	0.994 ± 0.001	0.990 ± 0.001	0.79 ± 0.12
3		15	0.992 ± 0.002	0.985 ± 0.001	0.67 ± 0.11
4		11	0.986 ± 0.001	0.975 ± 0.001	0.45 ± 0.04
5		6	0.960 ± 0.003		2.25 ± 0.3
2	2	19	0.995 ± 0.001	0.992 ± 0.001	0.82 ± 0.11
3		18	0.989 ± 0.002	0.980 ± 0.001	0.59 ± 0.10
4		8	0.985 ± 0.001	0.973 ± 0.001	0.52 ± 0.06
5		5	0.963 ± 0.002		2.12 ± 0.27
2	3	20	0.995 ± 0.002	0.991 ± 0.001	0.81 ± 0.12
3		16	0.990 ± 0.001	0,979 ± 0.001	0.64 ± 0.12
4		12	0.986 ± 0.001	0.975 ± 0.001	0.51 ± 0.05
5		4	0.960 ± 0.003		2.38 ± 0.3
2	averaged for the three kidneys	56	0.995 ± 0.002	0.991 ± 0.001	0.80 ± 0.12
3		49	0.990 ± 0.002	0.981 ± 0.001	0.63 ± 0.11
4		31	0.986 ± 0.001	0.974 ± 0.001	0.49 ± 0.05
5		15	0.961 ± 0.003		2.26 ± 0.3

Fig. 1. presents the results of ultrasonic velocity and absorption measurements in the longitudinal cross section of a kidney. It was found that there are five regions of kidney tissue which are acoustically distinct. It was not possible to make measurements at the boundaries of these regions because of high local heterogeneity of the tissue corresponding to the transition from one histological structure to another.

Fig. 2. shows the topographic sketch of the ultrasonic velocity and attenuation coefficient distribution in the longitudinal cross section of a dog kidney shown in the lower part of Fig. 2. The three dimensional images presented here are only the first, rough approximation to the real ultrasonic structure of a kidney.

The experimental results on the density, attenuation coefficient, ultrasonic velocity, acoustic impedance, and adiabatic compressibility distribution over the five regions shown in Fig. 1. were obtained from the kidneys of three dogs. These results are shown in Table 1. It can be seen that the absolute values of the measured parameters differ greatly for different kidneys. There are many possible reasons for this difference. The investigation of this matter is the subject of a separate study. For the purpose of medical imaging, it is the relative values of the acoustic charactersitics of tissue samples within one organ which are of importance. The relative values of the acoustic parameters of different regions of the investigated kidneys, compared to the corresponding value in the first region (Fig. 1.) of the same kidney, are shown in Table 2. It can be seen that the individual peculiarities of the different kidneys, which lead to the scattering of the individual measurements, does not influence the relative values of these quantities. Since this is, to our knowledge, the first paper describing the local ultrasonic properties of a kidney and its acoustic topography, it is difficult to compare these data with the literature values which were obtained using vastly different experimental conditions.

REFERENCES

1.   A.P. Sarvazyan, A high resolution and low volume method for tissue characterization, in "Abstracts of the 4th World Congress of Ultrasound in Medicine", Miyazaki, Japan (1979), p. 357.

COMPUTER-AIDED TISSUE CHARACTERIZATION OF THE HUMAN EYE

D. Decker, K.M. Irion and U. Faust

Institut für Biomedizinische Technik
Stuttgart
German Federal Republic

In the human eye the conditions for ultrasound diagnostics are very good because of the accessibility, the size and the regular structure of the organ. The detection of pathological changes in the tissue of the inner eye is even possible when the transparent parts of the eye are turbid and the common optical methods fail.

Accurate tissue differentiation requires an abundant acquisition of information on the interaction of ultrasonic energy with the tissue which is examined. This information is obtained from the RF-time-amplitude echogram. The analysis of these echograms requires computer-aided methods of evaluation in order to recognize tissue-dependent changes in the time, frequency and phase domains of the echogram[1,2,3,4,5].

For an objective tissue differentiation, knowledge of the tissue structure to be characterized is of crucial importance. Both the distance between the individual tissue boundaries, i.e. measurement of layer thicknesses, and a description of internal structures are required for such differentiation[6].

The method presented here is merely an acoustic method, which can be clinically applied and which does not require optical perception.

SIGNAL ACQUISITION

The examination of the patient is performed with a standard commercial system (OCUSCAN-400), to determine the region of interest. The signal is obtained by using a hand held, medium focused transducer with a frequency spectrum of 5...22 MHz; the nominal frequency is 15 MHz. When examining the eye, the doctor obtains a conventional video signal. In this representation he marks the echogram section, which should be transformed into computer compatible digital signals by means of a shiftable window of 2 μs. These digitized RF-echograms with a resolution of 9 bit are ready for computer-aided signal analysis on a mini-computer (PDP 11/40).

AUTOMATIC PREPROCESSING OF THE ECHOGRAMS

Quality Control

By means of various plausibility controls, disturbed signals are recognized and according to the degree of disturbance are restored or rejected. The number of rejected and restored echograms is registered.

The Formation of Patient Specific Representative Echograms

One or more representative echograms are constructed by means of controlled averaging in the time domain of echograms which are recorded from different areas of the tissue which is examined[7]. In this way the thickness of different layers, e.g. of membranes, or the mobility of tissue with blood vessels can be detected. To characterize the tissue, the number of representative echograms and the dispersion between each echogram and the averaged ones is used. Fig. 1. shows a preprocessed echogram of a detached retina.

SIGNAL ANALYSIS

In determining the distance of boundary surfaces we used various methods. The preprocessed signal was either analyzed visually, or autocorrelated, or cross correlated with a reference echogram obtained from a tissue-like reflector. Distance may also be measured by inverse filtering. The filter function is derived from the reference echogram mentioned above. To examine the retina, its echograms served as the input. The output signal shows maxima at a distance of Δt. With the known sound velocity c, the thickness of the retina can be calculated. If the echogram of a layered structure is transformed into the frequency domain, the result is a scalloping spectral distribution. From the constant distances Δf between the minima or maxima of the distribution, the distance of the reflectors can be determined by $\Delta s = c/(2\Delta f)$ with c = 1500 m/s.

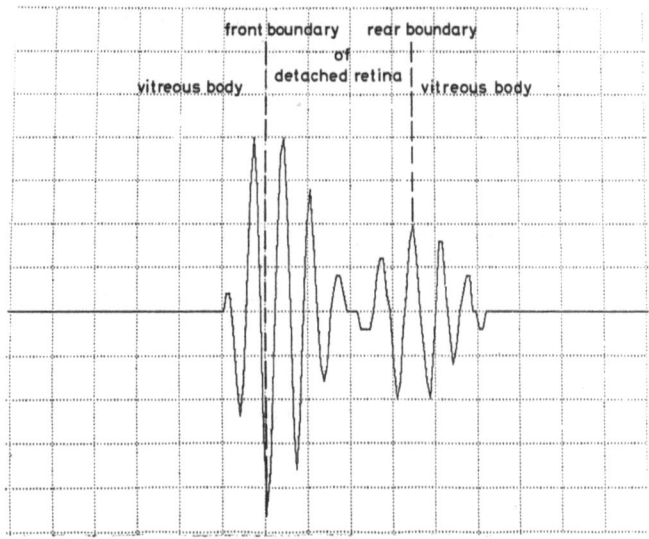

Fig. 1. Preprocessed signal (detached retina)

Apparently the methods seem to be similar, but it must be stated that the feasibility of the visual method is limited and that the routine application of inverse filtering involves much care.

The resolution and the accuracy by correlation and by spectral distribution have been compared. For reliable measurement of the layer thickness from the scalloping spectral distribution, at least four distinct minima are necessary. Hence, with an effective frequency range of 5...22 MHz there is an upper discrimination limit, $\Delta f < 6$ MHz, which corresponds with the smallest detectable layer thickness. Δs (min) = 125 μm.

In the clinical routine this optimum cannot be achieved. The applied transducer does not show an ideal Gaussian distribution in the frequency domain. Consequently, only layers of 180 μm and above can be measured by their spectral distribution.

For distances smaller than 170 μm we used the correlation method. The smallest layer thickness which can be measured with this method corresponds to the mean wave length λ of the ultrasonic pulse. For a center frequency of 15 MHz, Δs (min) = 60 μm is obtained.

For both methods the accuracy is given by the sampling rate of N = 256 for an echogram of 2 μs and by the actual echogram section (retina: 0.25 μs). In the case of 200 μm for a retina echogram, 33 sampling points are available for the correlation method, leading to an accuracy of 3% for this procedure. This applies for both the

autocorrelation and the cross correlation methods. With more than
two layers, only the cross correlation method can be applied. Due
to the sampling theorem the accuracy of the spectral method diminished
by the factor of 3 to 10%.

ANALYSIS OF BOUNDARY SURFACES

The analysis of the boundary surface is done in the frequency
domain by the spectral distributions (power spectra). According to
the roughness r of a surface related to the wave length λ, a
distinction is made between:

(a) Specular surface with $r \ll \lambda$ and a power spectrum similar to a
     Gaussian distribution. The reflected signal and its spectral
     distribution ($f_c \simeq f_N$), demonstrates the properties of the
     transducer.

     f_c : centre frequency of the distribution

     f_N : nominal frequency of the transducer

     r   : short-wave deformation of the surface shaping

(b) Scattering surface with $r < \lambda$ and with a homogeneous distribution
     of scattering elements. The spectrum of the reflected signal
     shows a single peak distribution with $f_c > f_N$.

(c) Structured surfaces with $r > \lambda$ and an inhomogeneous distribution
     of scattering elements. The spectrum shows a multi-peak or
     asymmetrical distribution.

SCATTER ELEMENTS WITH STOCHASTIC DISTRIBUTION

If the tissue does not reveal a layer structure but consists
of statistically distributed scatter elements (internal echoes of
tumors, haemorrhages etc.), the following must be taken into account:
A 2-µs-window of a haemmorhage or a tumor contains approximately
five structure elements (Fig. 2.).

The spectral distribution of such an echogram is not only
influenced by the frequency dependence of the tissue elements but
also by the distance of the scatter elements. This influence cannot
be completely eliminated by averaging of spectra recorded from
different positions. Our in vivo examinations of a multitude of
internal echoes showed that tissue-specific spectral attenuations,
which allow a reliable tissue differentiation, cannot be obtained
with this method. We therefore chose the following procedure.

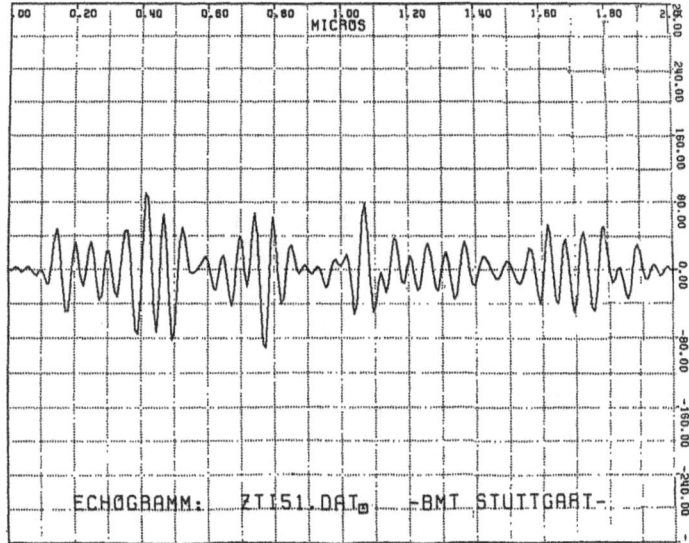

Fig. 2.   Internal echo

A special program tailored to the tissue-dependent structure
elements separates the individual scatter elements. The envelope
of the signal, which is calculated by special digital low-pass
filtering, contains peaks which are caused by the reflection of a
series of scatter elements. An algorithm detects minima and maxima
of the envelope. Another algorithm separates non-overlapping segments
which are delimited by the location of the envlope's minima. Each
segment is overlayed by a variable window function, (e.g. Hamming,
Hanning, Blackman, Bartlett). The window function, which is a good
compromise of design criteria, is the Hamming function (sidelobe
suppression). The set of segments are then transformed by FFT and
the power spectra are calculated. Attempting to reduce the number
of echoes to one for spectral analysis leads to short data segments.
Therefore, the true spectrum of one echo is modified or blurred by
shortening the length of the segments. We must then consider that
there are segments which are not too short and which all have
approximately the same length. In the 256-points dataset the
algorithm normally detects about seven segments for malignant melanoma, four segments for macula degeneration, and 3.5 segments for
membranes. Fig. 3. shows the averaged power spectra from segmented
echoes in the case of membranes (MEM), macula degeneration (MAC),
ablation (ABL), malignant tumors (TUO, TUIN), intact posterior wall
(RW), and in other cases.

A similar separation has been applied by Roman Kuc[8] for the
measurement of the slope of attenuation as the function of
frequency in the case of liver tissue. Our method differs in the
calculation of the envelope and minima detection of the envelope.

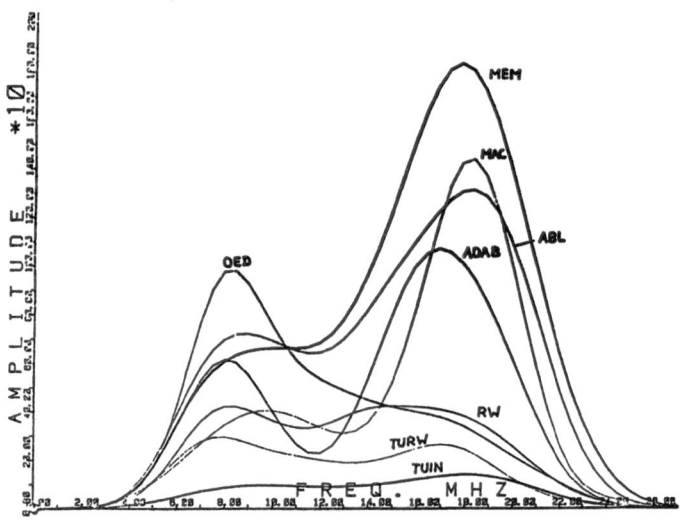

Fig. 3.   Power spectra

EXAMPLES OF TISSUE DIFFERENTIATION AND CHARACTERIZATION

Variance of Features

The variance of the features of boundary surfaces and their
dependence on the quality of signal acquisition (cooperation of the
patient, experience of the examiner) are shown in the following
examples. Table 1. shows the mean value and standard deviation of
the features of a detached retina for a patient collective (25 cases),
for a single patient with three spatially different recordings, and
for one recording consisting of 40 echograms.

Table 2. shows the mean value and standard deviation of the
features of malignant melanoma of the choroid and the intact posterior
wall. These collectives consist of 16 patients and 26 patients
respectively.

Set of Features for Boundary Surfaces

For each patient the features and their statistical properties are
are documented in the form of a patient's record. Fig. 4. shows a
section of this sheet.

Table 1. Mean value and standard deviation of the features of a
          detached retina

	Patient collective	Patient	Recording
Retina / μm	140 ± 10%	128 ± 13%	130 ± 7%
f_1 / MHz	11,5 ± 17%	10,5 ± 10%	14,0 ± 9%
f_2 / MHz	13,5 ± 25%	14,0 ± 12%	14,0 ± 9%

Table 2. Mean value and standard deviation of the features of
          malignant melanoma of the choroid and the intact posterior
          wall

	N = 16 Patient collective (malignant melanoma)	N = 1 Patient (malignant melanoma)	N = 26 Patient collective (intact post. wall)
Retina / μm	122 ± 15%	116 ± 20%	133 ± 18%
Second layer / μm	260 ± 30%	220 ± 38%	540 ± 21%
	(tumor component)		(choroid)
f_1 / MHz	13,5 ± 14%	14,6 ± 5%	12,6 ± 15%
f_2 / MHz	16,0 ± 10%	18.0 ± 2,5%	14,5 ± 14%
f_3 / MHz	17,0 ± 9%	18,5 ± 3,5%	13.0 ± 15%

f_1, f_2, f_3: Center frequency of the spectral distributions
              of the retina / choroid / sclera boundaries.

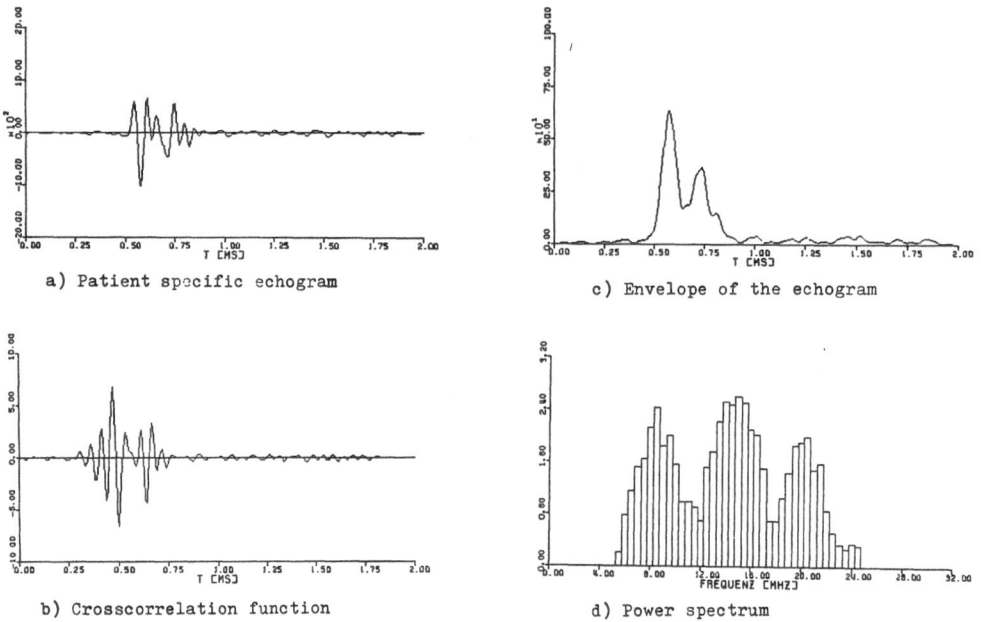

a) Patient specific echogram

c) Envelope of the echogram

b) Crosscorrelation function

d) Power spectrum

Fig. 4.   Patient's record

The upper left part contains a patient-specific averaged echogram (after preprocessing), of a serous ablatio. The cross
correlation function shown below is the result of correlating the
averaged echogram with the reference echogram. Layer distance and
phase reversal can be seen. The envelope of the echogram (top, right)
is to be compared with the video signal presuming the demodulator
is ideal. Below the spectral distribution (power spectrum) is
plotted, showing interferences distinctly. Table 3. contains the
significant properties for the characterization of the tissue layers
examined, such as distance and structure of the boundary surfaces
as well as data on the spatial inhomogeneity.

CONCLUSION

These examples demonstrate the working hypothesis of our research
group which postulates: A reliable characterization and differentiation of tissue demands an analysis in the time domain as well as
in the frequency domain of the tissue echogram. Only the compilation
of several features gathered from both domains of the signal may
yield a significant tissue characterization. This concept of signal
acquisition and evaluation allows the objective determination of
layers and also the structure of tissues with other organs, e.g. in
the abdomen, from the mammaries, or from the prostata.

Table 3

Boundary-surfaces	Features	Intact posterior wall	Macula* degeneration	Detached Retina	Choroidal* Haemangioma	Exudative* Inflammation	Malignant Melanoma (Type B)
1	occurence	100%	100%	100%	100%	100%	100%
	spectral distribut.	SP	SP	SP	SP	SP	SP
	centre freq./MHz	12,0	12,0	10,5	12,5	11,0	13,0
	reflectivity/dB	-20	-27	-28	-42	-16	-32
	boundary-dist./μm	133	100	128	0,90,120,160	120	122
11	occurence	100%	-	95%	-	-	100%
	spectral distribut.	SF	SP	SP	ST	SP	ST
	centre freq./MHz	14,5	14,0	14,0	16,5	13,5	15..18
	reflectivity/dB	-20	-27	-28	-42	-16	-32
	boundary-dist./μm	100	78	60..96..120	210	96	90
111	occurence	50%	*	25%	100%	*	60%
	spectral distribut.	SP	SP	SP	FS	SP	SP
	centre freq./MHz	13,6	13,6	13,6	(15,0)	10,5	14,5
	reflectivity/dB	-20	-27	-28	-42	-16	-32
	boundary-dist./μm	540	450-870			380	260
IV	occurence	50%	100%			100%	100%
	spectral distribut.	SP	SP			ST	FS,ST
	centre freq./MHz	14,0	14,0			17,5	17,0
	reflectivity/dB	-20	-27			-16	-32

*statistically not confirmed, N < 10 cases

Explanation	spectral distribution:	SP = specular surface
		ST = scattering surface
		FS = structured surface
	centre frequency:	centre frequency f_c of the spectral distribution with a nominal transducer-frequency of 15 MHz
	reflectivity:	in relation to a Kel-F-reference (15 mV $\hat{=}$ 0dB)

Set of features for boundary surfaces

ACKNOWLEDGEMENTS

This work was done in cooperation with H-C. Trier, R-D. Lepper and R. Reuter, Klinisches Institut für Experimentelle Ophthalmologie, Universität Bonn[9].

This project is supported by a research grant from the Bundesminister für Forschung und Technologie, Bonn, German Federal Republic.

REFERENCES

1. D. Decker, E. Epple, W. Leiss and M. Nagel, Digital computer analysis of time-amplitude ultrasonograms from the human eye II: Data processing, J. Clin. Ultrasound 1:156-159 (1973).
2. D. Decker, H-G. Trier, M. Nagel, R. Reuter, E. Epple and R.D. Lepper, Rechnergestützte Ultraschall-Diagnostik in der Ophthalmologie, in "Medizinische Physik, Bd. 2", W.J. Lorenz, ed., Dr. A. Hüttig Verlag, Heidelberg (1976).
3. D. Decker and K. Irion, A-mode RF-signal analysis (frequency domain), in "1st EEC Workshop on In Vivo Ultrasonic Tissue Characterization" (1979) (in press).
4. D. Decker, H-G. Trier, E. Epple, R. Reuter, M. Nagel and R-D. Lepper, Computer aided tissue differentiation in ophthalmology, in "Investigative Ultrasonology", C.R. Hill and C. Alvisi, eds., Pitman Medical (1980).
5. F.L. Lizzi, L. St. Louis and D.J. Coleman, Applications of spectral analysis in medical ultrasonography, Ultrasonics 14:77-80 (1976).
6. D. Decker and K.M. Irion, Examination of thin tissue layers, in "Fifth International Symposium on Ultrasonic Imaging and Tissue Characterization", Gaithersburg, U.S.A. (1980) (in press).
7. D. Decker, M. Nagel and W. Blocher, Rechnergestutze Gewebsdifferenzierung mit Ultraschall, Biomedizinische Technik 23:22 (1978).
8. R. Kuc, M. Schwartz and L. Micsky, Parametric estimation of the acoustic attenuation coefficient slope for soft tissue, in "Proceedings of IEEE Ultrasonics Symposium 76 CH 1120-5 SU: 44-47" (1976).
9. D. Decker and H-G. Trier, "Rechnergestützte Gewebsdifferenzierung' project of the Arbeitsgemeinschaft Bonn/Stuttgart Diagnostic Ultrasonica in Ophthalmologia, H. Gernet, ed., R.A. Remy-Verlag, Münster (1979).

SOFT TISSUE SIMULATION IN ULTRASONIC DIAGNOSIS

USING CROSS-LINKED HYDROPHOBIC GELS

P. Schuwert

Department of Radiation Physics
Karolinska Institute, S-104 01 Stockholm
Sweden

It is known that ultrasonic wave propagation and attenuation
in biological matter depends on density, macroscopic structure, and
viscoelastic properties such as the complex plane wave moduli
$M^+ = K^+ + 4/3\ G^+$, where K^+ and G^+ are the complex bulk and shear
moduli respectively[1]. In an attempt to identify suitable tissue
equivalent (TE) materials, an initial study of ultrasonic wave
propagation speed, and attenuation frequency power dependence, was
made on two hydrophobic gel systems. The influence of variation in
chemical structure, i.e. polymerization and cross-linkage degree,
was recorded in the frequency range 2-10 MHz including the effect
of introducing different scattering obstacles. Two different
measuring methods were used, wave amplitude transmission and a
modified resonance technique originally described by Eggers[2].

CHARACTERISTICS OF GEL MATERIALS

The study included the sonar characteristics of animal hide
based gelatine and aqueous acrylamide monomer, whose macromolecular
structure has been cross-linked by means of chemical reagents at
different concentration levels. The gelatine matrices were prepared
between 7.5% and 30% wet weight concentration (w/w) with a variation
in cross-linking degree using solutions of glutar-dialdehyde (GDA)[3].
In some samples glycerol and agar were added as speed and density
controllers. The acrylamide monomers were prepared at a 10% cross-
linking level with a monomer concentration between 10% and 40% w/w
to form a polyacryleamide (PAM) gel with a water content of 85-90%.
In those samples glycerol and agarose were also added (25-30% w/w
and 2.5-5% w/w respectively) to control speed and density variables
(Fig. 1.). Weak scattering ability of the gels, which increases

115

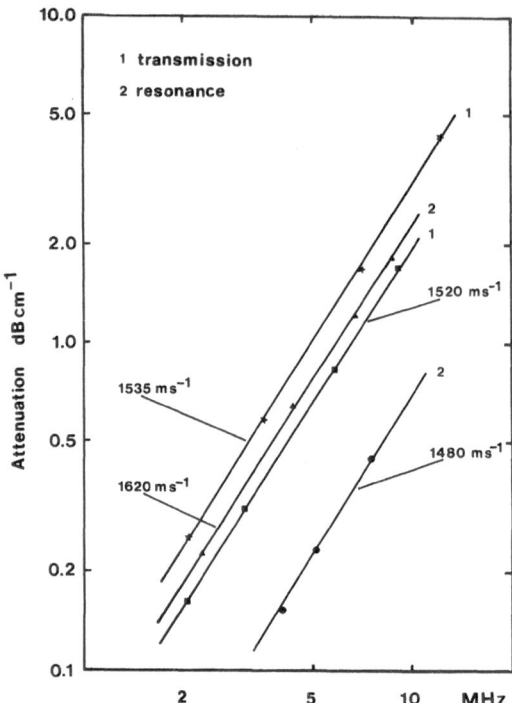

Fig. 1.   Attenuation frequency dependence.
          15% PAM, 30% Sephadex; 15% PAM, 20% PAM;
          20% PAM, 2.5% Agarose.

attenuation, was formed by the inclusion of sephacryl[4] microbeads
with an average diameter of 70 μm in the gel matrix before final
cross-linkage. A frequency power dependence of 0.05 $f^{1.5}$ was found
for those fluid simulating PAM-gels. Attenuation increased three-
fold with the inclusion of 30% sephacryl in a 15% PAM gel. Sound
speed (at 20°C) may be altered between 1480-1620 ms⁻¹.

Stronger scattering ability and much higher attenuation (relative
to water at 20°C) was formed by inclusion of obstacles consisting of
sephacryl beads, graphite or polyvinylacetate powder with dimensions
much less than a wavelength in the gelatine matrix (Figs. 2. and 3.).
The inclusion of scattering obstacles appears to lower the frequency
power dependence but increases the magnitude of attenuation (Fig. 3.).
Longitudinal phase velocity may be controlled with gel concentration
and to a lesser extent with cross-linking degree.

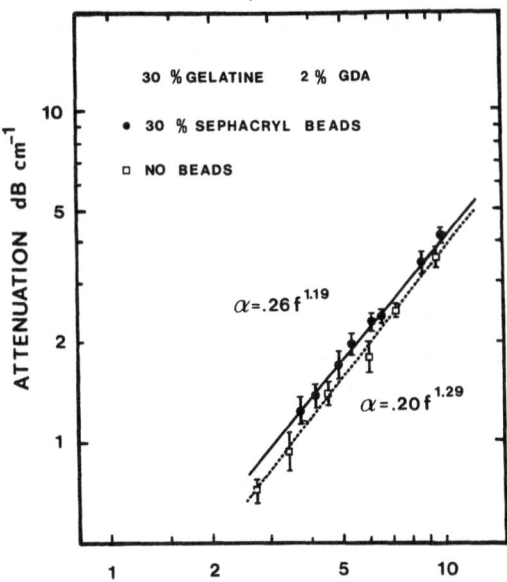

Fig. 2.   Frequency dependence of cross-linked gelatine.

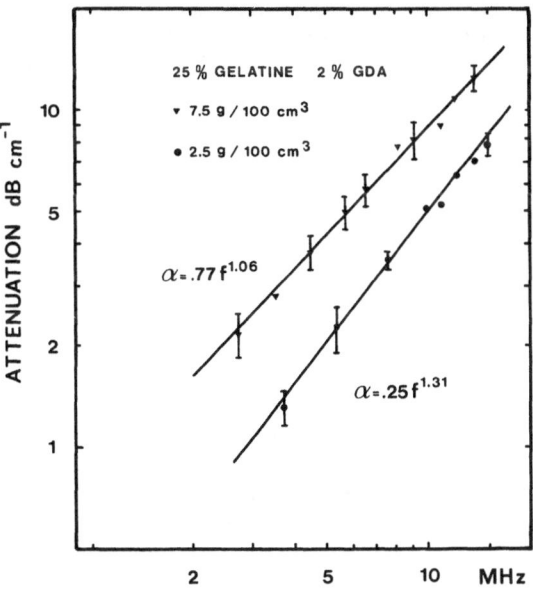

Fig. 3.   Frequency power dependence of gelatine with graphite
powders.

MEASURING METHODS

The amplitude transmission measurements were made with a set of 3.5 and 7.5 MHz broadband transducers as transmitters and a 0.5 mm^2 aperture hydrophone as a transceiver in the far field. Samples were molded between parallel glass plates, spaced by teflon rings of varying thicknesses, 5-20 mm.

Resonance measurements were made with 5 mm plane parallel sample discs placed in between two carefully matched 5 MHz transducers thus forming a resonating cell. Sound speed can be derived from the frequency jump between successive resonant peaks and the dimensions of the cell and the sample. Velocity determination was also made with a substitute technique described by Madsen and Zaqzebski[4] using a distilled water bath at 19-20°C as a reference. Agreement to within 1% was found for a gelatine matrix fixed with 2% GDA solution and the longitudinal wave speed ranges from 1500 ms^{-1} at 10% gel concentration to 1580 ms^{-1} at 30% concentration.

SUMMARY

The primary findings from both measuring techniques reveal a suitable attenuation frequency dependence (Figs. 1. to 3.), and easily altered sound speed (1480-1620 ms^{-1}) and density (1.01-1.10 g/cm^{-3}) properties. Introduction of isotropic weak to strong scattering centres increased the attenuation almost a magnitude indicating the relation between scattering power and total attenuation believed to consist of classical absorption together with relaxation phenomena and scattering/diffraction contributions[5].

ACKNOWLEDGEMENT

This study was supported in part by the National Swedish Board for Technical Development.

REFERENCES

1.   A. Matheson, "Molecular Acoustics", chapter 2, Wiley Inter-
        science (1970).
2.   F. Eggers, Eine Resonatormethode zur Bestimmung von
        Schallgeschwindigkeit und Dämpfung an geringen
        Flüssigkeitsmengen, Acustica 19:323-329 (1967/68).
3.   Private communication, Dr Rassing, Royal Danish Institute of
        Pharmacy, Copenhagen.
4.   E. Madsen and I. Zaqzebski, Med. Phys. (Oct. 1980).
5.   Dunn O'Brien, "Ultrasonic Bioacoustics" (1977)

ULTRASONIC BACKSCATTERING BY BLOOD

U. Cobet and A. Klemenz

Institute of Applied Biophysics
Martin-Luther-University
4014 Halle, Str. d. DSF 81
German Democratic Republic

Since the sensitivity and lateral resolution of ultrasonic pulse Doppler methods are restricted, continuous wave Doppler methods are introduced for examinations of relatively small vessels in the peripheral blood circulations. There are difficulties in the measuring of quantitative blood flow volume because an exact knowledge is necessary of the ultrasound scattering in blood by using continuous waves. Also, for the estimation of the mean velocity, it is necessary to know the distribution of frequency-dependent scattering from the velocity profile of blood flow.

However, blood has a relatively complicated structure and, due to this, the ultrasound interaction is not well known. Reid et al.[1] showed that the erythrocytes are mainly responsible for the formation of the signal of ultrasound scattering in blood.

However, due to a relatively high cell concentration of erythrocytes in a normal haematocrid value of about 45 per cent, and with the relatively long wavelengths of normal ultrasonic waves of frequencies of 4 to 10 MHz, we must assume that interference effects have a considerable influence. The mean distance from the erythrocyte surface to a neighboring erythrocyte surface is about 2 μm and the diffusion was estimated by the BOLTZMANN-MAXWELL relation to 0.3 μm/sec. Therefore it is not possible for the ultrasound scattering in blood with a high cell concentration to use the theory of Lord Rayleigh[2]. This has been seen in the experiments of Shung et al.[3].

An asymptotic approximation of single scattering for a small non-rigid sphere showed, according to Morse and Ingard[4], that the angle-dependent scattering of plane waves is proved by a change in density. A change in the ultrasound velocity produces spherical scattering waves, analogous to HYGHENS' principle and in contrast to scattering on a single rigid sphere.

According to Foldy[5] the total scattered wave from isotropic scattering by randomly distributed scatterers may be divided into two parts: the coherent and the incoherent. Whilst in the coherent part the amplitudes of the scattered waves interfere in definite phase with the transmitted signal; the incoherent parts summarize as an "intensity". Following the phase evaluation with the ultrasonic Doppler method from the received to the transmitted signal, we must assume from this relation that the coherent part is of considerable importance in the formation of the signal. According to Morse and Ingard[4] the coherent part completes the wave equation like a continuum and the scattered power is proportional to the square of N, the number of particles. In the power of the incoherent part we have a proportional relationship to N. With continuous waves and a high concentration of inhomogeneities the coherent part gains considerable importance, according to Glotow[6] and as discussed by Chivers[7], whilst with pulsed ultrasound the incoherent part increases.

From this, assuming that the blood behaves essentially as a continuum, we can conclude that ultrasonic scattering in the blood can only be carried out be geometrical inhomogeneities:

- inhomogeneities in the erythrocyte concentration;
- by the sound field geometry;
- by the geometrical dimensions of the blood vessel; or
- by a possible influence of the ultrasonic absorption into the blood.

An ultrasound goniometer was built for the experimental evaluation of the angle-dependent scattering, (Fig. 1.).

The experiment took place in the form of ultrasonic bursts on small blood-filled spheres. The geometrical dimensions of the goniometer were chosen in such a way that the blood sphere was in the farefield of the transmitter and that the receiver was in the farefield of the scattering sphere.

It could thus be arranged that the scattering is produced by plane waves and only one geometrical factor, the radius of the blood sphere, is introduced as an inhomogeneity. Long bursts were chosen in contrast to the diameter of the sphere.

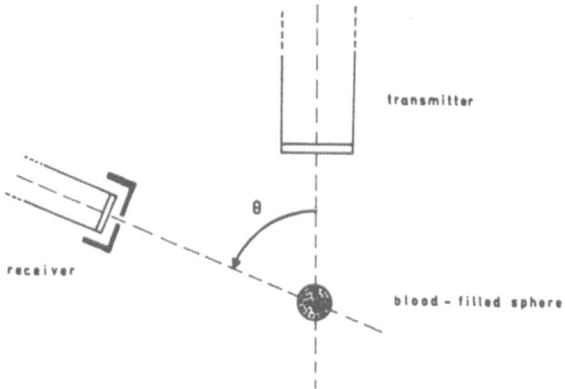

Fig. 1. Ultrasound goniometer for the measuring of angle-dependent
         scattering of ultrasound from a blood-filled sphere.

     Fig. 2. is the arrangement of the goniometer in our laboratory.
With the help of a thermostat we have the possibility to measure with
constant temperature. The blood-filled sphere is justified so that
we can interchange the blood over a very small tube in measuring
conditions.

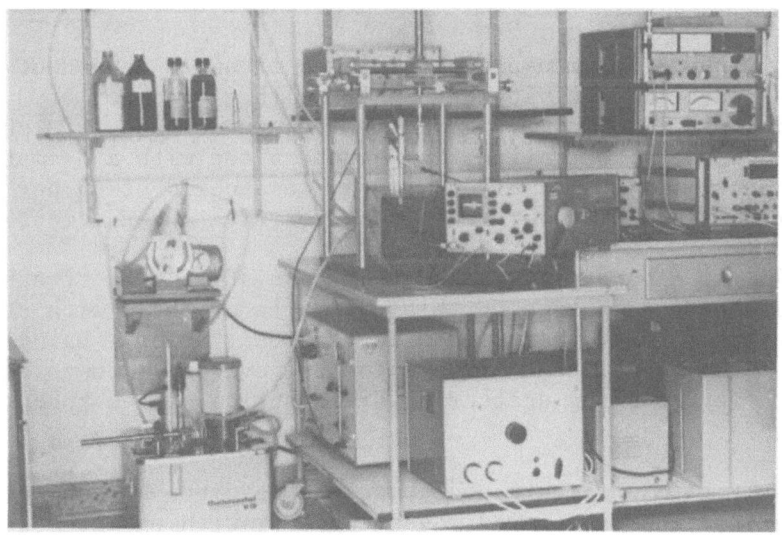

Fig. 2. Arrangement of the goniometer in the laboratory.

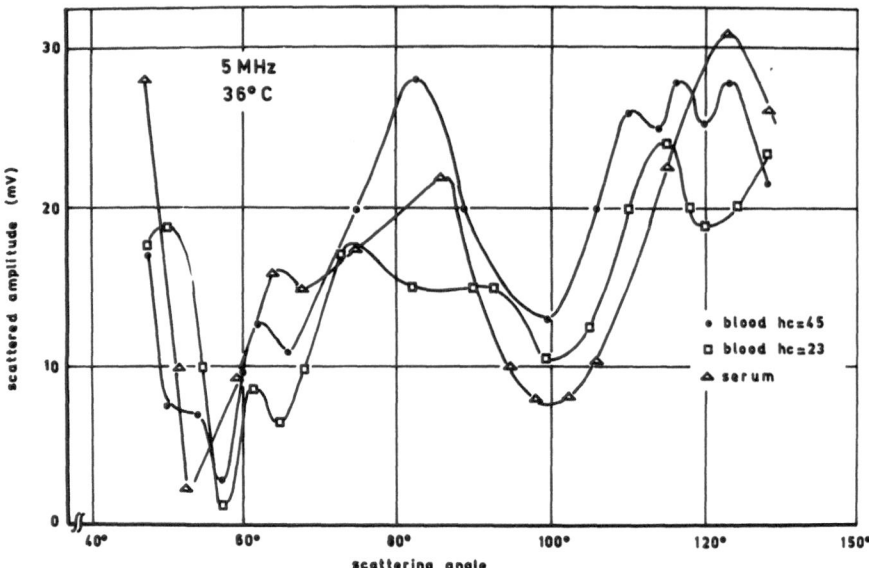

Fig. 3.   Angle-dependent scattering of a blood-filled polystyrene
          sphere with a diameter of 3 mm and a wall thickness of
          0.03 mm for human blood with a haematocrid of 45% (dark
          cycles) and 23% (open quadrangles) in comparison to serum
          (open triangles).

     Fig. 3. shows the measured amplitudes of angle-dependent scatter-
ing of a blood-filled polystyrene sphere with a diameter of 3 mm and
a wall thickness of 0.03 mm. In comparison three cases are shown,
the angle-dependent scattering from serum, blood with a haematocrid
of 23 per cent, and normal blood with a haematocrid of 45 per cent.
All measured points are average values over five observations.

     In Fig. 4. one can see the scattering distribution of a blood-
filled silicone rubber tube for blood, on the one hand with static
conditions and on the other hand with stationary flow. Using this
arrangement, no significant differences are evident. Compared to it
the thin curve shows the scattering distribution of the tube wall
alone.

     The initial experiments confirmed the assumption that the
coherent part of the scattered waves together with the geometrical
factors had a considerable influence on the scattering distribution
of blood vessels using continuous ultrasonic waves.

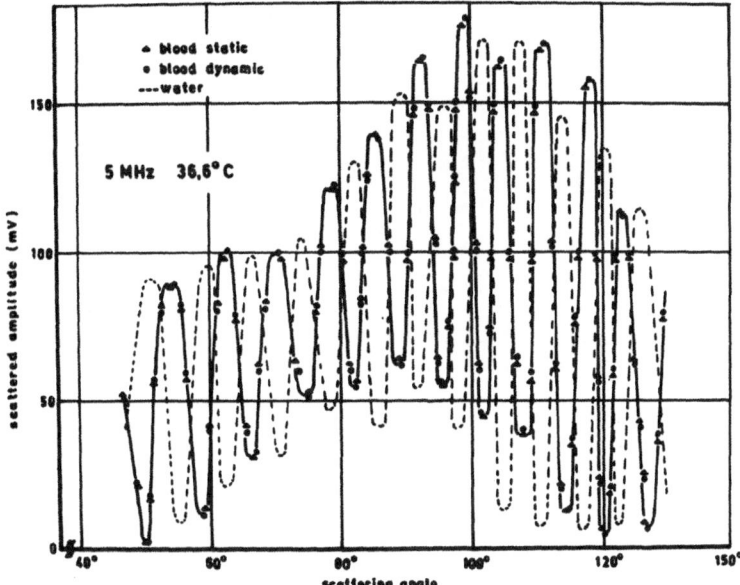

Fig. 4. Angle-dependent scattering of a blood-filled rubber tube
with a diameter of 3 mm and a wall thickness of 0.15 mm
with a haematocrid of 45% for static (triangles) and
stationary flow (circles) conditions by mean velocity of
10 cm/sec. in comparison to a water-filled tube.

REFERENCES

1. J.M. Reid, R.A. Sigelman, M.B. Nasser and D.W. Baker, The
      scattering of ultrasound by human blood, in Proceedings of
      8th I.C.M.B.E. (1978).

2. Lord Rayleigh, "Theory of Sound", Dover, New York (1945).

3. K.K. Shung, R.A. Sigelman and J.M. Reid, The scattering of
      ultrasound by red blood cells, Appl. Radiol. 77 (1976).

4. P.M. Morse and K.U. Ingard, "Theoretical Acoustics", McGraw
      Hill, New York (1968).

5. L.L. Foldy, Multiple scattering of waves: general theory of
      isotropic scattering by randomly distributed scatterers,
      Phys. Rev. 67:107 (1945).

6. V.P. Glotov, Coherent scattering of plane and spherical waves
      in deep water layers containing discrete inhomogeneities,
      Sov. Phys. Doklady 1:211 (1962).

7. R.C. Chivers, The scattering of ultrasound by human tissues:
      Some theoretical models, Ultrasound in Med. and Biol. 3:1
      (1977).

ULTRASONIC BACKSCATTERING IN BLOOD - BASIS FOR DOPPLER TECHNIQUES

H. Grossmann and A. Klemenz*

Research Institute M. von Ardenne, Dresden, GDR

*Institute of Applied Biophysics, MLU Halle, GDR

Pulsed doppler systems are used for instance to determine the blood flow velocity distribution along the diameter of a vessel (velocity profile).

The dopplershifted signal arises from the backscattering of the sound pulse at the moving particles (erythrocytes). The particle density in whole human blood is very high ($4.5 \cdot 10^6$ erythrocytes per mm^3). From this the mean distance between the erythrocytes is calculated to be about 10 μm. Supposing a pulse repetition frequency of 20 kHz and a blood flow velocity of 1 m/s the particles move between two pulses over a distance of 50 μm. Though every time another particle configuration scatters the sound, the mean received signal will not change due to the high particle density and because the radius of the scatterers is small compared to the wavelength.

At a fixed time t_o those signals attain the receiver, that are scattered in the so-called sample volume. The amplitude of this received signal may be evaluated as the sum of an exponential rising and decreasing sinusoidal function.

For the first case the sample volume may be completely inside the blood vessel. The received signal at the time t_o consists of differential parts, that are scattered at the time $t_o/2$ from the sample volume. These scattered signals interfere according to their phase conditions and the received signal may be calculated as integral of the scattered parts.

If the particle distribution is uniform, the time constants of the transmitted pulse are equal, the pulse consists of plane waves, and absorption losses are neglected, the received signal approaches zero (Equation 1).

125

$$\int_{0}^{5\lambda} (1 - e^{-\frac{x}{c\tau}}) \sin kx \, dx + (1 - e^{-\frac{5\lambda}{c\tau}}) \int_{0}^{\infty} e^{-\frac{y}{c\tau}} \sin ky \, dy = 0 \quad (1)$$

where $y = x - 5\lambda$

$c = $ velocity of sound

$\tau = $ rise and decrease time constant

$\lambda = $ wavelength

$k = \frac{2\pi}{\lambda}$

$x = $ distance

However, in most cases these assumptions are not met and so we receive a dopplershifted scattered signal with a small amplitude.

In pulse doppler systems the received signal is usually sampled for the time t_g. If we assume the gated signal to be the integral of the received signals during the time t_g, this signal also will vanish.

For the second case the sample volume may be partly inside and partly outside the blood volume. In this case only those parts of the transmitted pulse contribute to the received signal, that are scattered by the particles inside the blood volume. Under the assumption of the complete interference of the scattered signals the received signal has an amplitude that differs from zero considerably.

In conclusion: if a sound pulse is backscattered from a volume containing small particles in a dense distribution the received signal will vanish under the assumption that at the time t_0 the scattered amplitudes interfere completely. If the sound pulse is in the marginal zone, the received signal amplitude will rise considerably.

If we transfer these conditions to the signal processing in pulse doppler systems we find that the amplitude of the low frequency doppler signals depends on the location of the sample volume. Because of the high amplitudes in the marginal zone, it may be possible that these doppler frequencies will be overestimated. This further depends on the characteristics of the l.f. high pass filter and on the blood flow velocity in the vessel.

To verify this representation a simple experiment was carried out. We used a rectangular chamber that was bound with thin foils on two opposite sites. Fig. 1. shows the stimulating pulse and the received signals, when the ultrasound beam impinges normally to the foil.

Then the chamber was filled with water containing no scatterers and the angle of incidence was chosen to be 68°. No signals were received (Fig. 2.). If the chamber was filled with whole human blood we received high signal amplitudes at the times when the pulse enters and leaves the chamber (Fig. 3.).

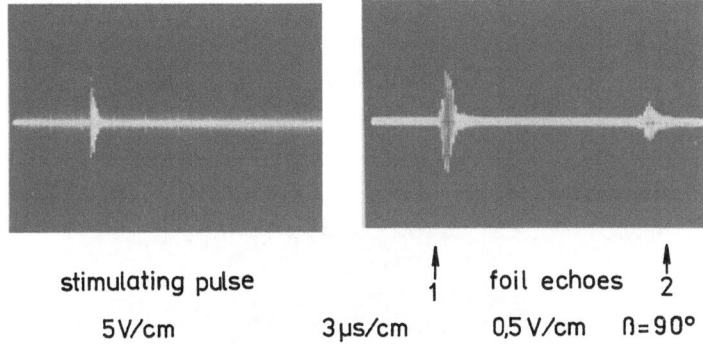

stimulating pulse   foil echoes

5V/cm   3µs/cm   0,5 V/cm   ß=90°

Fig. 1. Stimulating pulse and foil echoes (incident angle 90°)

We hope that the proposed wave interference representation will help to describe the backscattering of small pulses by blood, especially that it contributes to an explanation for the possible high dopplershifted signal amplitudes in the marginal zone of a vessel.

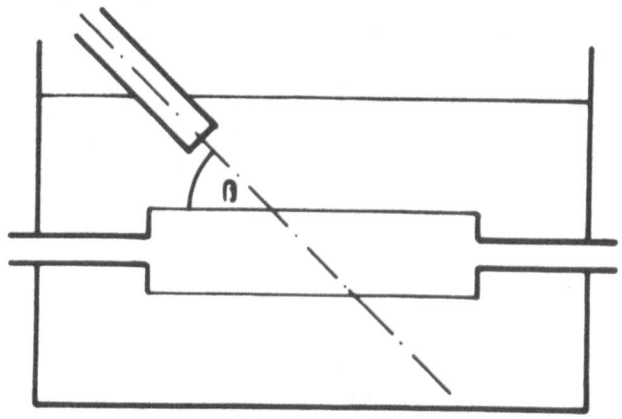

CHAMBER WITHOUT SCATTERERS

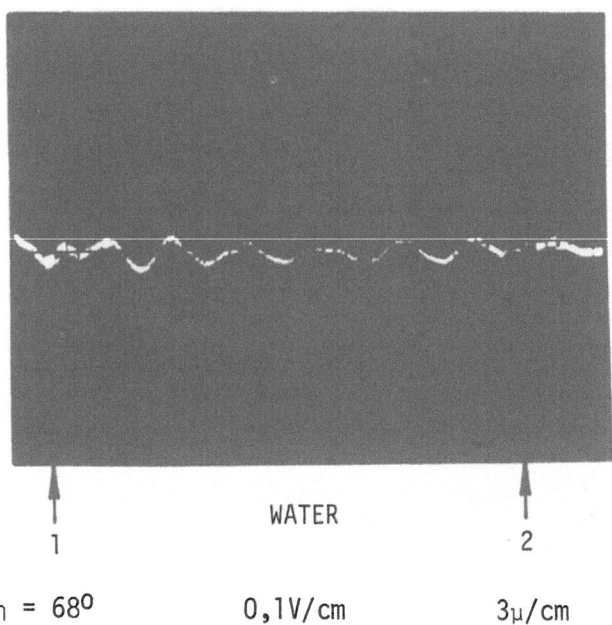

WATER

$\eta = 68^{o}$ 0,1V/cm   3µ/cm

Fig. 2.   Received signal from the chamber containing no scatterers
          (incident angle 68°)

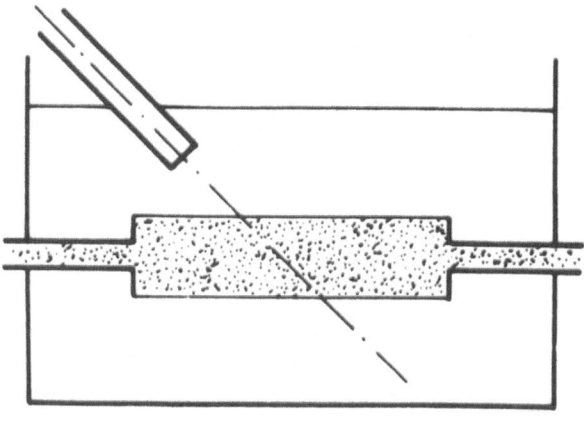

CHAMBER WITH SCATTERERS

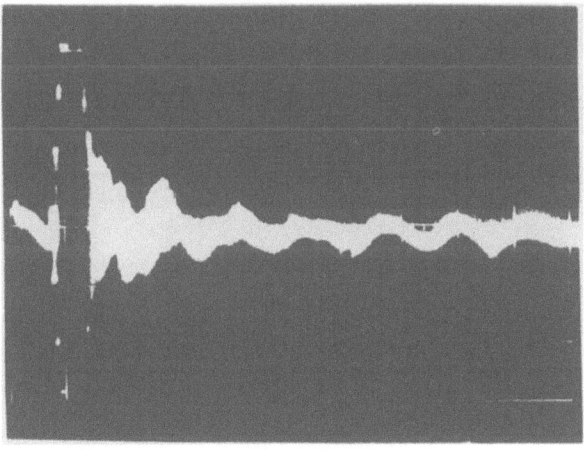

FLOWING BLOOD

Fig. 3.   Received signal from the chamber containing whole blood

PHYSICAL MECHANISMS FOR BIOLOGICAL EFFECTS

OF ULTRASOUND AT LOW-INTENSITY LEVELS

W.L. Nyborg and D.L. Miller

Physics Department
University of Vermont
Burlington, VT 05405
U.S.A.

INTRODUCTION: THE AIUM GENERALIZATION FOR MAMMALIAN TISSUES

Much of the recent increased interest in bioeffects of ultra-sound stems from the astounding success of ultrasound in diagnostic medicine. Because it is so widely used in examining pregnancies, it is now to be expected that much of the future population of the world will have been exposed to ultrasound before birth. As the societal impact of any environmental agent increases, so does public concern about its safety. Hence it is not surprising that questions are being raised from various quarters about possible risks from medical ultrasound, even though its safety record is excellent. It is necessary to respond to these questions now, and continuously, although most of us would very likely prefer to have more knowledge before passing judgements. In order to respond, a number of individuals and groups have turned to the scientific literature for help and have sought to form conclusions based on the published data. In Fig. 1. is a generalization arrived at by the Bioeffects Committee of the American Institute of Ultrasound in Medicine (AIUM). It was approved by the AIUM in 1976 and again, slightly revised, in 1978.

A number of comments accompanied the "AIUM Statement" when it was published and these deserve repetition:

1.   It is simply a generalization about scientific facts and hence, of course, is no more valid than the data on which it is based. The relevant data are still rather meager, especially for conditions typical of devices which use repeated short pulses. It is very possible that the Statement will have to be modified

131

as more information becomes available and, especially, when more
sensitive biological endpoints are considered.

2.   It does not, in itself, constitute a recommendation for medical
     practice. Specifically, the values cited for the exposure
     quantities, 100 mW/cm^2 for the intensity and 50 J/cm^2 for the
     intensity time product, are not necessarily to be taken as "safe
     upper limits"; as experience accumulates, it may turn out that
     higher values for these quantities are required for some
     applications, and are justified by the expected benefits. On
     the other hand, they are not necessarily "safe" values; it may
     be found in the future that lower values of the intensity and/or
     the intensity-time product should be used for some situations.

While the Statement was last approved in 1978, it appears that there
have been no results published since then that contradict it.
However, it applies only to experiments with mammals and, in fact,
is based mainly on experiments with small laboratory animals: mice,
rats, guinea pigs and rabbits.

STATEMENT ON MAMMALIAN IN VIVO ULTRASONIC BIOLOGICAL EFFECTS

August 1976:   Revised October 1978

     In the low megahertz frequency range there have been
(as of this date) no independently confirmed significant
biological effects in mammalian tissues exposed to
intensities* below 100 mW/cm^2. Furthermore, for ultrasonic
exposure times** less than 500 seconds and greater than one
second, such effects have not been demonstrated even at
higher intensities, when the product of intensity* and
exposure time** is less than 50 joules/cm^2.

* Spatial peak, temporal average as measured in a free field
  in water.

**Total time; this includes off-time as well as on-time for
  a repeated-pulse regime.

Fig. 1.   The "AMIUM Statement"

BIO-EFFECTS AT "LOW INTENSITIES"

Other experiments have shown that under some conditions bio-logical systems are affected by ultrasound at values of the intensity or the intensity-time product lower than those indicated in the AIUM Statement and, sometimes, in ranges commonly used in diagnostic medicine. These experiments were not with in vivo mammalian tissues, but instead dealt with the kinds of situations listed in Table 1. Some of the experiments referred to in this table were done with pulsed equipment such as is used in diagnosis. For this the characteristic time-averaged intensity is "low" in the sense used here; we note that it is the time-average which is referred to in the Statement of Fig. 1. However the intensity during a pulse is much larger, typically, by a factor of the order of 10^3.

In discussing some of the experiments on which Table 1. is based, we shall keep in mind the question: "Why should these systems be affected at lower values of the exposure quantities than are required for the mammalian systems to which Fig. 1. applies?"

Item (a) in Table 1. refers partly to experiments done with leaf tissue of the water plant Elodea. For this tissue it is known[2,3] that gas is contained in long intercellular channels with cross-sectional dimensions of about 5-10 microns. A theory for resonance properties of such cylindrical gas-filled spaces, with elastic walls, was developed by D.L. Miller[4] and compared with experimental results[5]. In a typical leaf there were two sizes of channels and the computed resonance frequencies fell into the two ranges (0.5-1.0 MHz and 2-4 MHz) shown by bars near the frequency axis in Fig. 2. Plotted in the same figure are results of experiments in which the Elodea leaves were exposed to ultrasound at various frequencies and at various intensities, and observations made on many cells in order to determine the threshold for cell death as a function of frequency. (Here "threshold" is defined as the spatial peak intensity which results in disrupted, or dead, cells in 50% of

Table 1. Biosystems affected by "Low Intensity" ultrasound

(a) Plant tissues;

(b) Cell cultures and cell suspensions;

(c) Cell suspensions in the presence of hydrophobic material with gas-filled pores; and

(d) Insect larvae.

---

the exposed leaves.) The threshold curve shows two minima which seem
to correspond to the two ranges of computed resonance frequency; the
match is particularly good for the lower minimum. This correspondence
gives very strong support for the influence of intercellular gas
channels in mediating damage of these plant cells by ultrasound at
low intensities. The evidence was made even more convincing by tests
showing that when leaves were centrifuged to remove the gas, the
intensity required for cell damage was greatly increased. In obtaining the data of Fig. 2. the exposure time was 100 s. and it is
therefore clear that the smallest intensity-time products required
for cell death were less than 50 J/cm^2. Also the lowest intensity
threshold in Fig. 1. is well below 0.1 W/cm^2. Furthermore, in
similar experiments using 10 s. pulses and a repetition period of
10 ms. the time-averaged spatial peak intensity was only 11 mW/cm^2.

Other experiments with Elodea and with Vicia faba roots were
carried out by Martin et al.[6]. These authors used a commercial
doppler fetal heart detector (Sonicaid) which generates and ultrasonic beam of frequency 2.1 MHz with total power output of 7.0 mW,
the average intensity over the transducer face being calcualted as
2.9 mW/cm^2 under free-field conditions. They used an arrangement
which allowed them to subject leaf tissue to the ultrasound while
the leaf was simultaneously under view with light microscopy.
(Unavoidably, the system also led to standing waves, as pointed out
by the authors.) They made quantitative studies of rotational

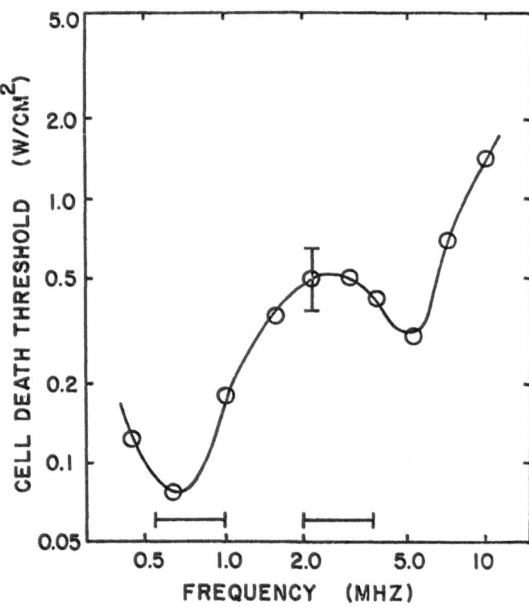

Fig. 2. Evidence for resonant response of gas-filled channels in
         Elodea. From reference (5).

movements of chloroplasts in the cells and found that the fastest
rotation occurred among groups of organelles on the edges of cells
adjacent to gas-filled channels.

Extensive studies have been made by Carstensen, M.W. Miller and
associates at the University of Rochester, in which roots and other
plant tissues were subjected to ultrasound at frequencies in the
1-5 MHz range; representative publications are cited[7,8]. Among
their findings were changes in growth patterns, reduction in mitotic
activity and chromosome aberations. While the intensities employed
were usually 1 W/cm^2 or more, the intensity-time products required
to produce significant biological change were frequently very small,
viz., only a few joules per square centimeter. In explaining their
results these authors attach considerable importance to cavitation-
like activity and, especially, to the oscillations of gas-filled
intercellular spaces. However, they also cite evidence for other,
as yet unidentified, mechanisms.

Item (b) in Table 1. refers to experiments in which ultrasound
is applied to suspensions of cells in aqueous media. There have
been several reports of biological change produced by diagnostic
ultrasound in this kind of situation. A recent paper by Liebeskind
et al.[9] is an important example. The use of suspensions as test
systems offers many advantages but also poses difficulties; perhaps
chief among these are uncertainties about the extent to which cavitation occurs. In the megahertz frequency range the gaseous bodies
or "nuclei" which act as sites for cavitation are no larger than a
few microns in diameter, and are not easily detectable. The state
of nucleation in a suspension may well determine the outcome of a
sonication experiment; unfortunately, it can usually be neither
measured nor controlled and it is probably very different in vitro
than it is in the animal body. This problem led to the experiments
discussed next.

In category (c) are experiments[10,11] carried out at the
University of Vermont in order to address the question: "How will
low-intenisty ultrasound affect cell suspensions in the presence of
known distributions of gaseous nuclei?" It is not easy to control
nuclear populations but an approach was made by the use of special
hydrophobic membranes which contain straight-through pores of
controlled size. When these are immersed in aqueous media, air
remains in many of the pores which then become the desired "nuclei".
Thus in an ultrasonic field any gas-filled pore may be the site of
vigorous activity. The gaseous body trapped there has dynamical
characteristics, including resonance properties, similar to those
for a free spherical bubble. In the membranes we have used, there
are about 1000 pores per square milimeter, with diameter three to
four microns. When a strip of this membrane is immersed in cell
suspension and exposed to an ultrasound field, each trapped gaseous
microbody responds with volume pulsations, its resonance frequency

being in the megahertz range. These pulsations lead to a number of phenomena, some of which are as expected from principles of physical acoustics[12]. Thus radiation forces cause cells to move towards and collect at active pores, while acoustic streaming and radiation torque produce eddying in the fluid and twisting of cells and organelles[10].

When a suspension of platelet-rich-plasma is sonicated in this way, the platelets gather around active pores and are subjected to stresses there. Irreversible clumping has been found to occur, using ultrasound from a widely used commercial fetal monitor[11]. Associated with this is the release of intracellular constituents including ATP. By using a photometric method, Williams and Miller[13] have been able to demonstrate directly, for red cells as well as platelets, that ATP is released from cells by ultrasound at low-intensity levels if suitable gas-filled pores are present. From red cells free ATP is detected at spatial peak intensities as low as 20-30 mW/cm^2, and from platelets at even lower levels.

Item (d) refers to a very recent report by Carstensen and others[14] in which they find that pulsed ultrasound with character-istics typical of commercial diagnostic devices is damaging to larvae of Drosophila. They show that the high intensity which occurs during each pulse is more critical than the time-averaged intensity, and suggest a cavitational mechanism involving the gas-filled respiratory channels in the larvae.

CONCLUSIONS

We return now to the list of situations in Table 1. for which bioeffects of ultrasound have been reported at low-intensity levels. In categories (a) and (c) the importance of gas-filled spaces has been established. In (d) gas spaces have been implicated and in (b) there is a general suspicion that most effects are caused by some form of cavitation. A conclusions seems warranted: low-intensity ultrasound is especially likely to produce change if gas-filled pores, crevices, bubbles, etc. are present. It is for this reason that many (if not all) of the experiments represented by Table 1. show bioeffects at relatively low values of the exposure parameters.

It is not known how to relate this conclusion to the situation for mammalian tissues (Fig. 1.) where significant bioeffects have not been demonstrated convincingly except at higher values of the exposure quantities. Future investigations will probably shed light on the matter.

Some of the research reported here was supported by the National Institutes of Health via Research Grant GM-08209.

REFERENCES

1. AIUM Bioeffects Committee, brochure entitled "Who's Afraid of of a Hundred Milliwatts per Square Centimeter?" available from American Institute of Ultrasound in Medicine, 4405 East-West Highway, Suite 504, Washington, D.C. 20014.
2. E.N. Harvery, E.B. Harvery and A.L. Loomis, Further observations on the effect of high frequency sound waves on living matter, Biol. Bull. 55:459 (1928).
3. A. Gershoy, D.L. Miller and W.L. Nyborg, Intercellular gas: its role in sonated plant tissue, in "Ultrasound in Medicine, Volume 2", D.White and R. Barnes, eds., Plenum Press, New York (1976), pp. 501-511.
4. D.L. Miller, A cylindrical-bubble model for the response of plant-tissue gas bodies to ultrasound, J. Acoust. Soc. Am. 65:1313-1321 (1979).
5. D.L. Miller, Cell death thresholds in Elodea for 0.45-10 MHz ultrasound compared to gas-body resonance theory, Ultrasound in Med. & Biol. 4:351-357 (1979).
6. D.J. Martin, H.G. Gemmell and D.J. Watmough, A study of streaming in plant tissue induced by a doppler fetal heart detector, Ultrasound in Med. & Biol. 4:131-138 (1978).
7. M.W. Miller and G.E. Kaufman, Effects of short-duration exposures to 2 MHz ultrasound on growth and mitotic index of Pisum sativum roots, Ultrasound in Med. & Biol. 3:27-29 (1977).
8. E.L. Carstensen, S.Z. Child, W.K. Law, D.R. Horowitz and M.W. Miller, Cavitation as a mechanism for the biological effects of ultrasound on plant roots, J. Acoust. Soc. Am. 66:1285-1291 (1979).
9. D. Liebesking, R. Bases, F. Elequin, S. Neubort, R. Leifer, R. Goldberg and M. Kuenigsberg, Diagnostic ultrasound: effects on the DNA and growth patterns of animal cells, Radiology 131:177-184 (1979).
10. W.L. Nyborg, A. Gerhoy and D.L. Miller, Interaction of ultrasound with simple biological systems, pp. 19127 in "Ultrasonics International 1977 Conference Proceedings", IPC Science and Technology Press Ltd, Guildford, England.
11. D.L. Miller, W.L. Nyborg and C.C. Whitcomb, Platelet aggregation induced by ultrasound under specialized conditions in vitro, Science 205:505-507 (1979).
12. W.L. Nyborg, "Physical Mechanisms for Biological Effects of Ultrasound", HEW Publications (FDA) 78-8062, Bureau of Radiological Health, Rockville, MD 20857.

13. A.R. Williams and D.L. Miller, Photometric detection of ATP
     release from human erythrocytes exposed to ultrasonically
     activated gas-filled pores, Ultrasound in Med. & Biol.
     6:351-256 (1980).
14. S.Z. Child, E.L. Carstensen and S.K. Lam, Effects of ultrasound
     on Drosophila: III Exposure of larvae to low-temporal-average·
     intensity, pulsed irradiation, Ultrasound in Med. & Biol.
     (1981, in press).

CAVITATION THRESHOLDS IN BIOLOGICAL TISSUES

V.B. Akopyan

Moscow Veterinary Academy
Scriabina 23
109472 Moscow, USSR

The problem of cavitation and its thresholds in biological tissues is one of the main problems in investigating the mechanism of biological action of ultrasound. In the megacycle range of ultrasound frequencies cavitation in viscous -- from 0.25 to 1.0 P -- biological media was for a long time supposed to arise only at sufficiently high intensities of ultrasound[1], (of the order of 10-100 W/cm^{-2}).

However, "holes" discovered by Curtis[2] on thin cuts of liver and other tissues, as well as weak noise at the frequency of the first subharmonic registered by Hill[3] in tissues at the intensity of about 1 W/cm^{-2} can be estimated as indications of cavitation. Apart from that, Gavrilov showed that cavitation thresholds for the focused ultrasound in tissues were not more than twice that of tap water[4]. If this relationship is also valid for the plane wave, then cavitation in tissues may be expected to appear at an intensity of ultrasound of about 0.6 W/cm^{-2}, since the theoretical threshold of cavitation in water is approximately equal to 0.35 W/cm^{-2}. At this intensity the acoustic pressure reaches 1 atmosphere. The thresholds measured experimentally in water at the frequency of 1 megacycle are in good agreement with the theoretical values[5].

Besides the characteristic noise, sonoluminescence and the formation of hydrogen peroxide, nitric and nitrous acids, OH-radicals etc. may be considered the main signs of acoustic cavitation in water media saturated with air. Yet measuring the sonoluminescence intensity in optically dense animal tissues is difficult while the identification of the substances formed in the ultrasound field is practically impossible. This is due to the small concentration of these substances and their high chemical activity.

Our investigations have been carried out on potato tuber tissue. This tissue has a cell structure and approaches animal tissues by acoustic parameters. Along with this it is sufficiently transparent. This allows the sonoluminescence intensity in it to be measured. In addition if a potato tuber is presaturated with luminol solution which on reacting with hydrogen peroxide gives a characteristic blueish-green luminescence one can register the effect of the formation of chemically active particles in the tissue, irradiated by ultrasound. There is also nothing to prevent one registering acoustic noise in the tissue of potato tubers.

For this purpose it is convenient to use a miniature ceramic hydrophone. In our experiments sonoluminescence and sonochemi-luminescence were registered by means of a simple instrumentation, (Fig. 1.). A plate of potato tissue was placed on a flat ceramic transducer. A photoelectron multiplier sensitive in the range of 350-650 nm was used as a photodetector.

Measurements were carried out on the samples of various thicknesses and it was discovered that the dependence of sonoluminescence upon thickness is of a periodical character, with the periodical equal to half wave length (Fig. 2.). The amplitude of these periodic changes decreases with the increase of the sample thickness, evidently due to the absorption of ultrasound energy. Apparently, the periodicity points to the appearance of standing waves in the sample. However, the notion of ultrasound intensity was introduced for the plane traveling wave and is meaningless for the standing wave. The notion of the intensity of ultrasound irradiation, which is, by the way, most commonly used, characterizes the irradiator. It also characterizes the ultrasound intensity in the medium near the irradiator in ideal cases. It is convenient to characterize both a travelling and a standing wave by the magnitude of variable acoustic pressure. In a traveling wave this pressure is connected with ultrasound intensity by a well-known relationship,

$$p \approx 10^{-3} \sqrt{2 \, \rho \, cI} \; .$$

The acoustic pressure in loops of a standing wave is twice the pressure amplitude in the original traveling waves.

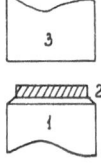

Fig. 1. Experimental arrangement.
          1. Transducer; 2. Sample; 3. Photomultiplier.

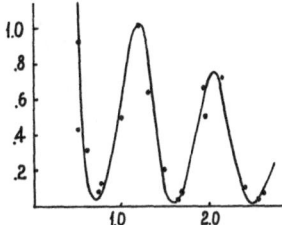

Fig. 2.   The dependence of sonoluminescence upon thickness of
          samples.

For example: the cavitation threshold in water corresponds to
1 atmosphere of variable acoustic pressure. For a running wave it
corresponds approximately to 0.35 W/cm^{-2} while for a standing wave
it is about 0.1 W/cm^{-2} of the original running wave.

Standing waves seem to arise rather often in experimental and
clinical conditions. For instance, when irradiating a rabbit helix,
human and animal muscle layers liquid in cuvettes and so on. In all
these cases the character of ultrasound waves should by all means
be taken into consideration. In Fig. 3. is shown the dependence of
the sonoluminescence intensity (in relative units) of the samples
of potato tuber tissues of the same thickness (curve 1) and the
dependence of sonochemiluminescence of samples saturated with luminol
solution (5 mg luminol and 50 mg soda in 100 ml of water) upon the
intensity of ultrasound irradiation (curve 2).

Sonoluminescence appears at the intensity of ultrasound
irradiation of 0.3-0.4 W/cm^{-2} and increases with the further increase
of intensity.

At the same threshold values, luminol chemiluminescence appears
in potato tuber tissue (curve 2). The fact that the dependence upon
ultrasound intensity is a little more abrupt than that for sonoluminescence appears to be due to the increase of activity of
peroxidase in the potato tuber under the action of ultrasound[6].
This leads to the acceleration of decay peroxides accumulating in
tubers in storage.

The character of the dependence of tissue luminescence upon
the ultrasound intensity is similar to the analogous dependence for
water and water solutions[7]. Evidently, in both cases the same
mechanism caused by cavitation takes place. Weak acoustic noice
also appears in potato tuber tissue at the intensity of about
0.3 W/cm^{-3} and along with sono- and chemiluminescence points to the
appearance of cavitation. Comparing the data mentioned above with
the obtained dependence of threshold of sonoluminescence appearance
upon the viscosity of glycerine solutions[5] one can see that the
cavitation threshold in potato tuber tissue and in solutions with
the viscosity of 0.25 P are approximately equal.

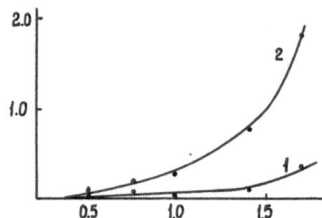

Fig. 3.   Intensity of sonoluminescence (1) and sonochemiluminescence
          (2) of potato tuber tissue as functions of ultrasound
          intensity.

As pointed out above, according to some estimates the viscosity
of cytoplasma may considerably exceed this value and reach 1 P.

However, the tissue heterogeneity, the presence of ions in them,
macromolecules and so on that diminish the cavitational durability
of the medium can contribute to the decrease of the cavitation
threshold in tissues. The same effect is achieved by a reversible
decrease of the viscosity of cell contents under the action of
ultrasound of quite small intensities.

The cavitation threshold in animal tissues seems to be a little
higher than that in plants, since plant cells contain vacuoles filled
with liquid of small viscosity. Still the difference in thresholds
seems to be slight and cavitation in animal tissues accompanied by
sonoluminescence, formation of chemically active particles, shock
waves and energetic microstreamings appears at intensities used in
therapy and leads to considerable biological effects.

REFERENCES

1.   I.E. Elpiner, ed., "Ultrasound" (in Russian), Nauka, Moscow (1973)
2.   J.C. Curtis, Effect of ultrasound on tissues and organs, in
         Interaction of Ultrasound and Biological Tissues", J. Reid
         and M. Sikov, eds., DHEW publ. (1972) pp. 115-118.
3.   C.R. Hill, Detection of cavitation, in "Interaction of Ultrasound
         and Biological Tissues", J. Reid and M. Sikov, eds., DHEW
         publ. (1972) pp. 199-200.
4.   L.P. Gavrilov, Physical mechanisms of the destruction of bio-
         logical tissues with focused ultrasound (in Russian),
         Akusticheski zhurnal 20, I:27-32 (1974).
5.   A.I. Zhuravlev, V.B. Akopyan, eds., "Ultrasound Luminescence"
         (in Russian), Nauka, Moscow (1977).
6.   O.K. Istomina, E.P. Ostrovski, Effect of ultrasound on the growth
         of the potato (in Russian), Doklady AH SSSR, new series, 1
         vol. 9 (1935), pp. 632-633.

7.   M.A. Margulis, V.B. Akopyan, Experimental investigations on sono-
     chemical reaction rate and sonoluminescence intensity in
     dependence upon the intensity of high power ultrasound (in
     Russian), Zhurnal fizicheskoi khimii 52 vol. 3 (1978),
     pp. 601-604.

MORPHOLOGICAL AND FUNCTIONAL STUDY OF THE ULTRASONIC EFFECTS

ON THE GOLDFISH MAUTHNER CELL

T.N. Pashovkin, P.V. Mashkin,
D.A. Moshkov, and A.P. Sarvazyan

Institute of Biological Physics
Academy of Sciences of the USSR.
Pushchino, 142292, USSR

The action of ultrasound on morphological and functional states of identified central neurons -- Mauthner cells (M-cells) -- was investigated. M-cells are the pair of giant neurons in the fish medulla oblongata. They receive the numerous synaptic endings from vestibular apparatus, through acoustic nerve branches[1]. M-cells innervate contralateral spinal motoneurones, which in turn govern the tail and body muscles. M-cells play a definite role in the modulation of fishes' swimming activity, being intercalating neurons in the otolyths-musculature pathway. The latter point of view has been confirmed by numerous experimental data[2,3].

The purpose of this study was to determine the short term functional changes in irradiated M-cells providing that non-specific reaction of tissue had not yet developed. An attempt was made to reveal the neuronal structures responsible for specific reaction to ultrasound. Obviously any structural changes in M-cells must be reflected in animal behaviour due to interneuronal connections of M-cells.

MATERIALS AND METHODS

The irradiation of the M-cells area in the goldfish brain was produced by a therapeutic T-5 generator at the frequency of 880 KHz and the spatial average intensities within the range of $0.1-1.0$ W.cm^{-2}. The intensity was estimated by the radiation force measurements. Total time of exposure was varied from 15 seconds to 20 minutes. The fish was fixed in the special thermostated chamber at the distance of 1 cm in front of the ultrasonic transducer.

The irradiation was performed at a temperature of $18^{\circ}C$. The temperature in the chamber was measured before and immediately after irradiation. The functional state of M-cells was estimated using a special quantitative test by automatic registration of the goldfish behavior in a ringshaped chamber[4]. The following criteria were used to describe behavioral changes of the sonicated fish:

(a)   changes in general swimming reaction, determined by the speed of the fish, and

(b)   changes in the turning reaction determined by the number of turns the fish makes in the measuring chamber.

Morphological changes in M-cells were examined with an electron microscope JEM-100B after conventional procedures of fixation, embedding and ultrathin sectioning of the appropriate nerve tissue.

RESULTS

1.   Behavioral test indirectly reflecting changes in functional state of M-cell after exposure to ultrasound is shown by:

   (a)   Irradiation for 30 sec. at intensities of 0.1 $W.cm^{-2}$ produced no effect, irradiations for 5 min. increased the swimming activity of goldfish by 10-20% and 10 min. exposure increased the activity by up to 150%.

   (b)   Irradiation for 30 sec. at intensity of 1.0 $W.cm^{-2}$ resulted in depression of the swimming activity by 20-30% from the control values. This depression was reversible and completely disappeared in 10 min.

   (c)   The 5 min. exposure at an intensity of 1.0 $W.cm^{-2}$ resulted in a 70-80% decrease in the activity which was slowly restored within 30-40 min. A second 5 min. irradiation at an intensity of 0.1 $W.cm^{-2}$ resulted in the immediate restoration of depressed activity.

   (d)   Irradiation for 10 min. at 1.0 $W.cm^{-2}$ produced a partially reversible 100% depression of the swimming activity and 20 min. exposure resulted in complete and irreversible behavioral depression followed shortly after by the death of the fish.

2.   Ultrastructural analysis has shown that the sonication of M-cells by intense ultrasound (1 $W.cm^{-2}$) for 10 min. and more resulted in destructive changes in mauthnerian apparatur ultrastructure, visible more prominently in myelin sheaths of their presynaptic

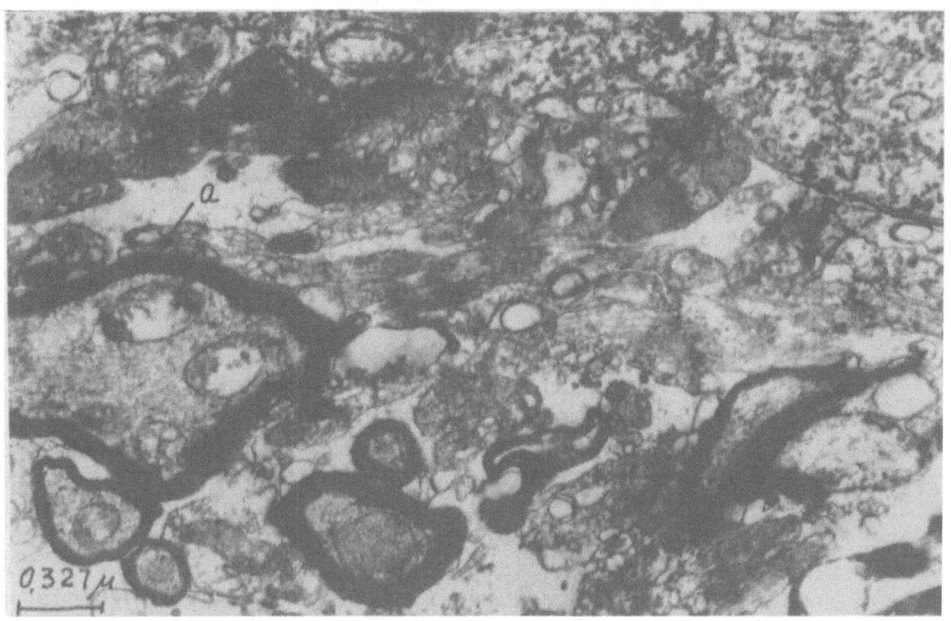

Fig. 1. Ultrastructure of the Mauthner cell, control.
(a) myelin sheaths

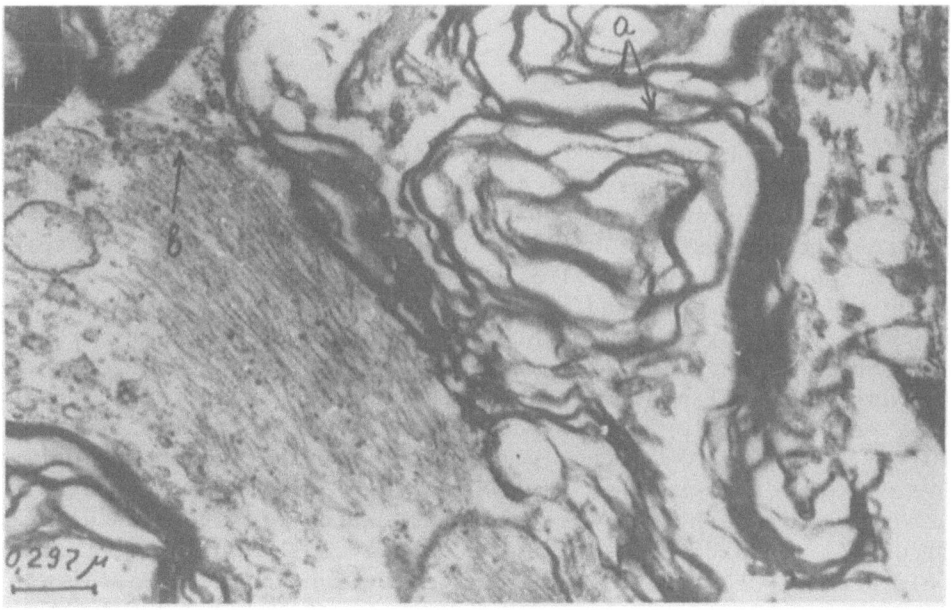

Fig. 2. Destructive changes in Mauthnerian apparatus ultrastructure.
(a) in myelin sheaths;   (b) in axolemmas.

fibres and also in axolemmas. Probably as a consequence, the full depletion of the M-cells axosomatic synapses, and total disappearance of the synaptic vesicles was revealed, (Fig. 1, Fig. 2).

These morphological data correlate with sharp and irreversible behavioral immobilization of the goldfish in a ring-shaped chamber, thus indicating a decrease of M-cells function after treatment by high intensities of ultrasound (1 $W.cm^{-2}$). Ultrasound did not produce visible destruction of the myelin sheaths or axolemmas of presynaptic fibres, upon being applied for 5 min. or less, but induced drastic changes in the M-cells' cytoplasm. These alterations consisted of dense, crystalline structures within the M-cells' perikaryon, (Fig. 3).

The crystal-like structures might be of neurofilament origin since simultaneous disappearance of those within the cytoplasm occurred. Besides, deep invaginations and evaginations of the nuclear envelope took place in this case. The latter presumably indicated the changed nuclear-cytoplasmic relationship. It was of interest to note that if immediately after such high, damaging irradiation the fish was sonicated by low intensity ultrasound (0.1 $W.cm^{-2}$ for 5 min.), the crystalline structures disappeared and the cytoplasm ultrastructure became nearly normal, including the pattern of cytoplasmic neurofilaments, (Fig. 4).

This was in good correlation with the goldfish behavior being returned to control values immediately after treatment by ultrasound of low intensity.

DISCUSSION

It is well known that low intensities of any external physical factor, including ultrasound, induce stimulating, activating effects in biological systems, while high intensities inhibit or destroy the object. The intensities of ultrasound generally used in therapeutic applications vary within 0.1-1.0 $W.cm^{-2}$. Physical mechanisms for biological action of ultrasound can be completely different at the limits of this intensity range. At the upper limit of this range many different physical phenomena such as local temperature increase, various mechanical processes and even cavitation can take place in the irradiated biological object[5]. At the lower intensities ($10^{-2} - 10^{-1}$ $W.cm^{-2}$), probably the main contribution to the primary physical processes in the ultrasonic field comes from mechanical factors, having a hydrodynamical nature, from different unidirectional forces[5]. This difference in the nature of the acting mechanisms could probably be responsible for the observed differences in the character of ultrasonic biological effects at 0.1 and 1.0 $W.cm^{-2}$.

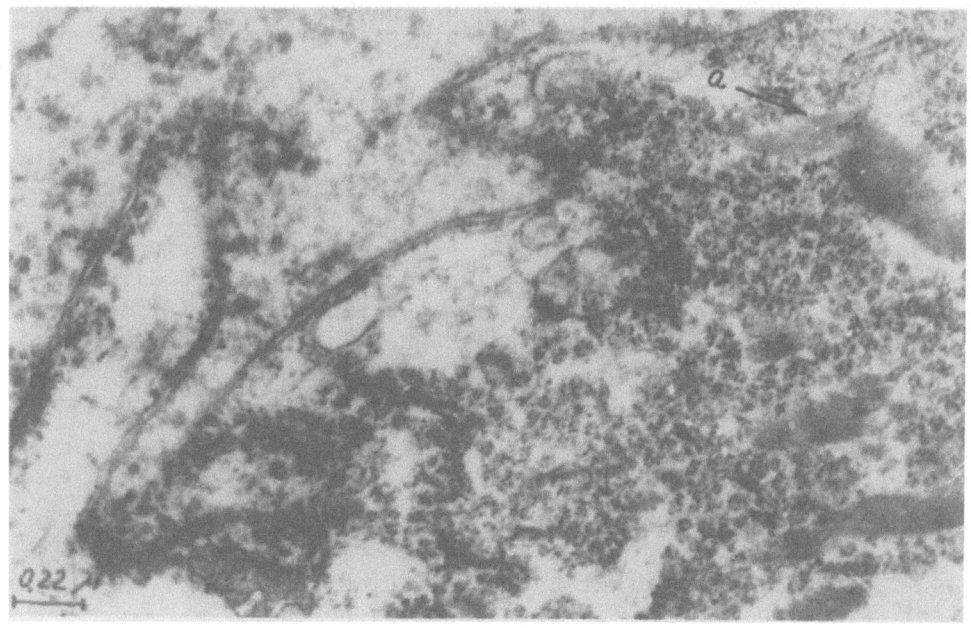

Fig. 3. Ultrastructure of the Mauthner cell after 5 min. sonication
         by ultrasound at the intensity of 1.0 W.cm^{-2}.
         (a) crystalline structures

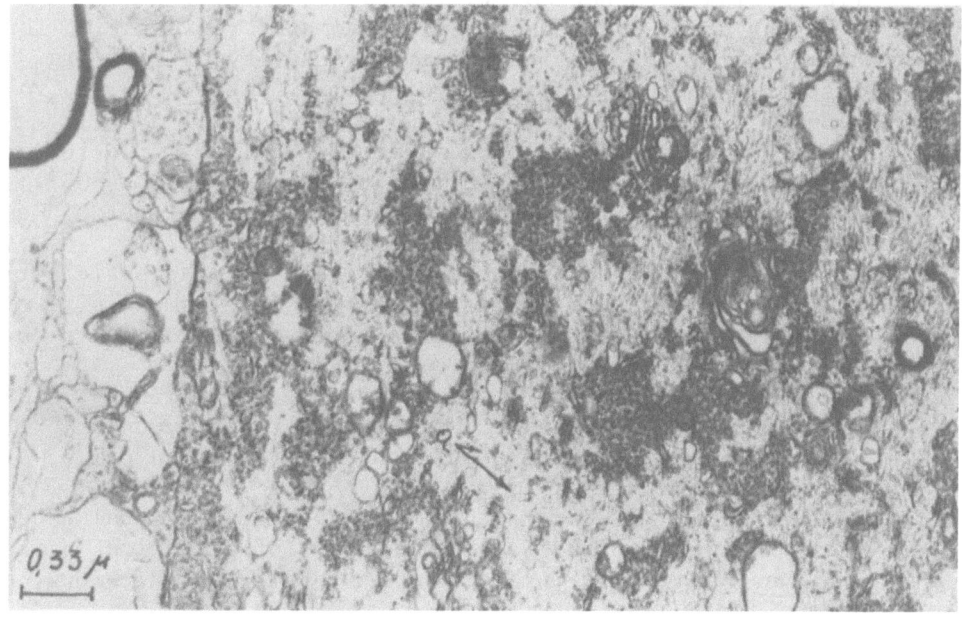

Fig. 4. Ultrastructure of the Mauthner cell after 5 min. sonication
         by ultrasound at the intensity of 0.1 W cm^{-2}.
         (a) neurofilaments

Most of the experimental data presented in literature and used for estimation of the threshold for ultrasonic bioeffects are related to structural changes in sonicated objects[6].

Only recently some papers describing functional effects of low intensity ultrasound started to appear[7,8,9]. Usually the stimulating action of ultrasound is detected by indirect tests or delayed effects. It is a difficult problem to show immediate structural changes in the biological object exposed to low intensity ultrasound. Experiments presented in this paper show not only functional effects of low intensity ultrasound, but also provide immediate direct registration of the morphological changes responsible for the functional effects. Electron micrographs clearly demonstrated quick restoration of the normal cell ultrastructure after irradiation by 0.1 W.cm^{-2} intensity, after having been damaged by 1.0 W.cm^{-2} ultrasound shortly before.

REFERENCES

1. J. Diamond, The Mauther cell, in: "Fish Physiology", Academic Press, New York, (1971), volume 5, p. 265.
2. S.J. Zottoli, Comparison of Mauthner cell size in teleosts, J. Comp. Neur., 178:741 (1978).
3. L.I. Sasyuk, D.A. Moshkov and S.B. Terekhova, Behaviour of goldfishes in a ring-shaped chamber by vestibular stimulation and the ultrastructures of Mauthner cells (in Russian), in "Ultrastructure Investigations of the Plasticity of Neurons" (in Russian), Pushchino (1981), p. 20.
4. L.I. Masyuk and D.A. Moshkov, Half automatic registration for quantitative tests of the movement activity of fish (in Russian), Zhurnal evolyutsii biokhimii, fisiologii 16, vol. 3: 318-319 (1980).
5. W.L. Nyborg, "Physical Mechanisms for Biological Effect of Ultrasound", HEW Publ. (FDA) (1978), volume 78, p. 8062.
6. I.M. Reid and M.R. Sikov, eds., "Interaction of Ultrasound and Biological Tissues", DHEW Publ., Wahington (1973).
7. N. Murai, K. Hoshi and N. Nakamura, Effect of diagnostic ultrasound irradiated during fetal stage on development of orienting behaviour and reflex ontogeny in rats, Tokyo J. Exp. Med., 116:17-24 (1978).
8. E. Siegel, J. Goddard, E. James and P. Siegel, Cellular attachment as a sensitive indicator of the effects of diagnostic ultrasound exposure on cultured human cells, Radiology, 133:175 (1979).
9. M.R. Sikov, B.P. Hildebrand and J.D. Stearns, Postnatal sequelae of ultrasound exposure at fifteen days of gestation in the rat, in "Ultrasound in Medicine", D. White and R. Brown, eds., Plenum Press, New York (1977).

EFFECTS OF ULTRASOUND ON WOUND CONTRACTION *

M. Dyson and D.S. Smalley

Anatomy Department
Guy's Hospital Medical School
London SE1 9RT, England

Wound contraction is the reduction of part or all of a skin defect by centripetal movement of the surrounding undamaged skin[1]. It plays an important part in wound healing, the restoration of continuity in living tissue, since it reduces the size of the tissue defect. The edges of the lesion move inwards and the stretched healthy skin beyond the lesion responds by interstitial growth. Wound contraction appears to be brought about by the shortening of linked myofibroblasts and to be maintained by the deposition of collagen fibers in the granulation tissue which develops at the wound site.

Ultrasonic therapy can stimulate skin repair[2,3] and experimental evidence suggests that it should stimulate the contraction part of the process. For example, contraction of nonstriated myocytes (smooth muscle cells) can be induced by treatment with therapeutic levels of ultrasound[4]; since these cells have much in common with myofibroblasts, both structurally and functionally, it might be expected that the latter would respond in a similar way. Indeed, it has been suggested that myofibroblasts may actually be smooth muscle cells, formed by the differentiation of local fibroblasts in response to injury[5].

---

* This investigation was supported, in part, by the National Fund for Research into Crippling Diseases (Grant Number A/8/1017).

The possibility that ultrasound might affect wound contraction
was investigated in the following matter. Cryosurgical lesions of
equal surface area were made through the full thickness of the right
and left flank skin in male rats (Wistar, 225 ± 12 g.) anaesthetized
with fluothane. The lesions were made with a cryosurgical probe
(Spembly, Ltd.) cooled to -50°C by rapidly expanding gaseous nitrous
oxide. The probe was pressed into 1 ml. of KY Jelly (Johnson &
Johnson) encircled by a perspex ring of 1 cm. diameter, placed on
the shaved flanks of the animals. The KY Jelly ensured good thermal
conductivity, while the ring helped to limit the size of the resulting
lesion. The probe was held in this position for 30 seconds to obtain
cryo-adhesion, and then raised to lift the skin clear of the body
wall, thus avoiding damage to the underlying organs. Freezing was
continued for a further 2.5 minutes to complete lesion production.
The lesions corresponded in area to that of the interior of the
perspex ring. The epidermis, dermis and the panniculus carnosus,
a layer of striated muscle fibers deep to the dermis, were all damaged
by the cryosurgical procedure, but the underlying musculature of the
body wall was not involved. An example of a typical cryosurgical
lesion is shown in Fig. 1.

Once the lesions had been produced, 8 regularly-spaced Indian
ink tattoo marks were made in the undamaged skin around the circum-
ference of each lesion, within 2 mm. of the area of skin which showed
marked erythema after thawing. As Fig. 1. shows, the boundary of
the lesion is at first clearly defined. Changes in the area of the
defect can be measured from tracings and photographs for the first
14 days after injury, after which time the boundary of the lesion
becomes indistinct, and the linear displacement of the tattoo marks
gives a more reliable measure of wound contraction. One lesion from
each rat was treated with ultrasound immediately after operation and
the contralateral lesion was mock-irradiated as a paired control.
Ultrasound was delivered from a Rank-Sonacel Multiphon generator at
a frequency of 3 MHz and at a space-averaged intensity of 0.5 W/cm^{-2},
pulsed 2 ms on and 8 ms off for a total of 5 minutes, contact between

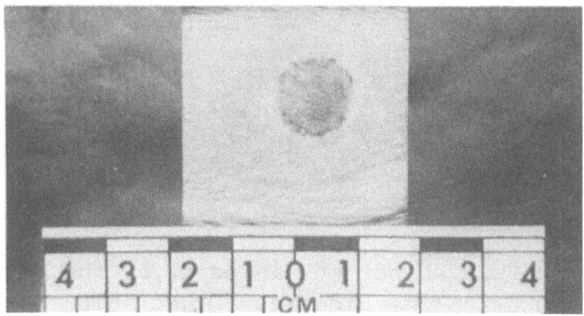

Fig. 1.   Surface view of a cryosurgical lesion made in the flank
          skin of a rat.

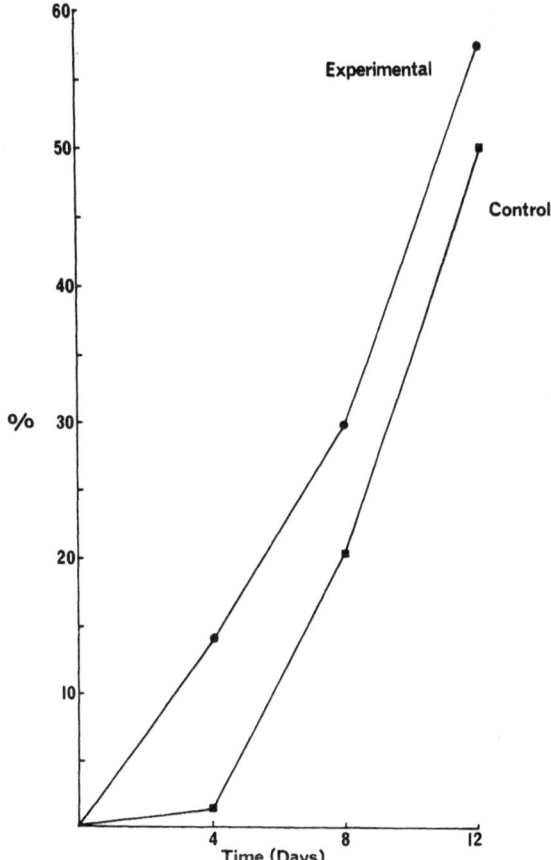

Fig. 2.   Decrease in wound area expressed as a percentage of the
          initial lesion area. Each point of the graph is the mean
          of 6 results.

the applicator face and the skin being maintained by means of a thin
film of Halas Coupling Cream (Rank Stanley-Cox). The applicator
face, which had a surface area of 7.55 cm^2, was moved over the lesion
and the adjacent undamaged skin throughout the treatment period,
thus reducing the time of exposure of local cell groups to the peak
intensities of the field and avoiding the production of standing
waves. Mock-irradiations were conducted in a similar manner but
without the production of ultrasound. A total of 8 treatments were
given, separated by 48 hour intervals. The effect of this procedure
on wound area is shown in Fig. 2. and Table 1.

       Comparison of the differences in contraction between the experi-
mental and control lesions of each animal by means of a student's
paired t-test showed that there was significantly more contraction
in the experimental lesions than in the controls at 4 and 8 days
after injury ($p<0.0$. and $p<0.05$ respectively). Although the experimental lesions continued to show more contraction than the controls
at 12 days, the difference between them was no longer significant.

Table 1. Effect of ultrasound on percentage decrease in wound area

			Days after wounding			
	4		8		12	
Specimen Number	Exp (+US)	Con (−US)	Exp (+US)	Con (−US)	Exp (+US)	Con (−US)
1	11.7	4.7	23.2	14.3	65.8	65.5
2	13.6	−0.7	30.9	20.9	53.1	39.9
3	22.6	0	30.5	19.2	38.4	27.6
4	15.5	1.3	27.3	9.7	68.5	54.0
5	12.1	−0.7	36.0	23.8	51.4	50.0
6	7.0	3.6	28.1	33.7	62.5	62.2
Mean	13.7	1.5	29.3	20.3	56.6	49.9
$\pm$ SE	2.1	0.9	1.8	3.4	4.6	5.8
Student's paired t	4.6		2.8		2.4	
p	< 0.01		< 0.05		NS	

Abbreviations: Exp (+US) = Experimental wound, treated with ultrasound

Con (−US) = Bilateral control wound, mock-irradiated

SE = Standard error of mean

NS = Not significant

More information on the effect of ultrasound on wound contraction was obtained when the linear displacement of the tattoo marks was followed over a longer period. Change in the mean linear displacement of diametrically opposite tattoo marks is shown in Fig. 3. and Table 2.

The first indication of there being more contraction in the experimental untrasonically-irradiated lesions than in the mock-irradiated controls was found 4 days post-operatively, a result in general agreement with that obtained by direct measurement of surface area. It is noteworthy that this was followed by a second increase in contraction rate in the ultrasonically-treated lesions and that this increase continued beyond the last irradiation (given on the fourteenth day). The biphasic nature of the contractile response to

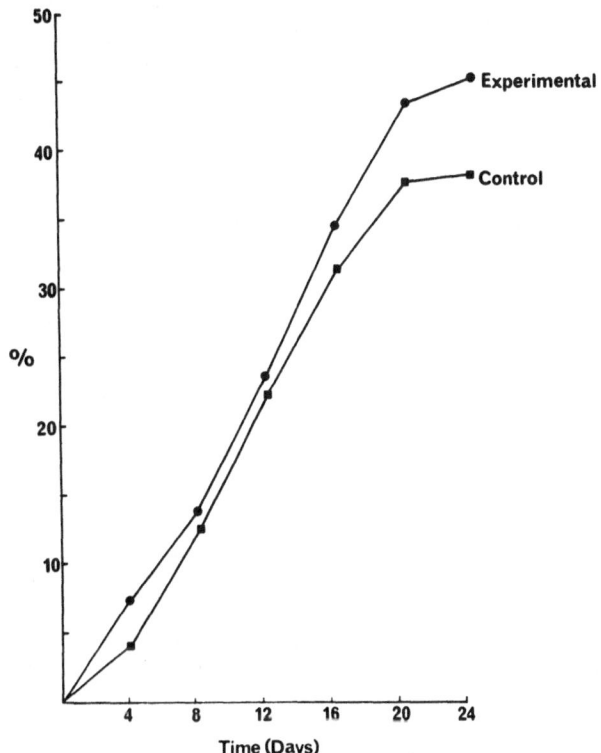

Fig. 3. Decrease in separation of diametrically opposite tattoo
marks, expressed as a percentage of their initial separation.
Each point on the graph is the mean of the pooled results
obtained from 6 lesions.

ultrasound is brought out particularly clearly if contraction of
each experimental lesion is expressed as a fraction of contraction
in the contralateral control lesion, as in Fig. 4.

Table 2. Effect of ultrasound on the percentage decrease in linear
          displacement of diametrically opposite tattoo marks.

	Days after wounding					
	4		8		12	
Specimen Number	Exp (+US)	Con (-US)	Exp (+US)	Con (-US)	Exp (+US)	Con (-US)
1	10.7	8.2	18.5	18.8	32.9	29.8
2	9.1	6.7	15.5	15.8	29.5	23.2
3	10.7	7.8	15.5	14.4	18.2	15.2
4	7.3	2.8	13.5	9.9	33.3	30.0
5	1.3	-1.1	9.5	8.2	17.8	17.6
6	6.5	0.8	12.2	9.4	15.4	21.1
Mean	7.6	4.2	14.1	12.7	24.0	22.8
$\pm$ SE	1.4	1.7	1.3	1.7	3.2	2.5
Student's paired t	4.36		2.11		0.82	
p	<0.01		NS		NS	

	Days after wounding					
	16		20		24	
Specimen Number	Exp (+US)	Con (-US)	Exp (+US)	Con (-US)	Exp (+US)	Con (-US)
1	40.0	37.2	42.1	37.9	---	---
2	36.6	30.0	48.0	39.1	49.6	41.4
3	28.6	21.5	36.8	30.3	39.7	34.8
4	43.8	39.9	47.3	44.2	47.5	39.2
5	---	---	---	---	---	---
6	28.1	28.6	---	---	---	---
Mean	35.4	31.4	43.5	37.9	45.6	38.5
$\pm$ SE	3.1	3.3	2.6	2.9	3.0	1.9
Student's paired t	2.88		4.41		6.37	
p	<0.05		<0.05		<0.05	

Abbreviations: as in Table 1.

           --- = Position of tattoo marks unclear.

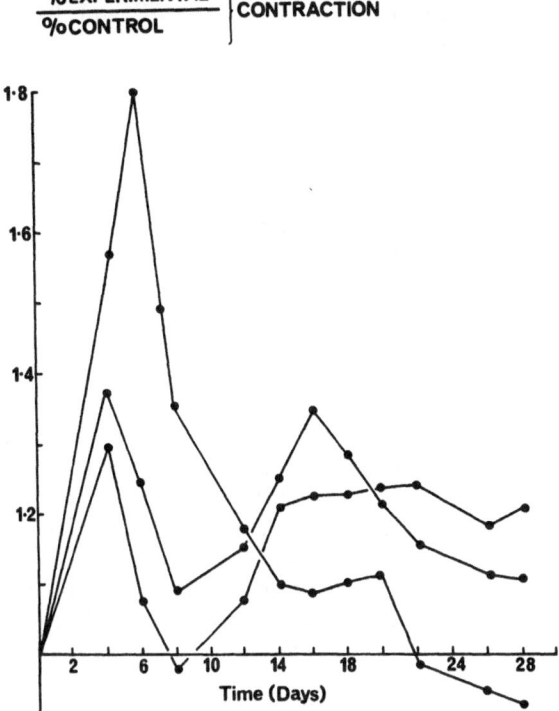

Fig. 4.   Biphasic nature of the contractile response of skin wounds
          to ultrasound. A point higher than 1 on the Y-axis indicates
          stimulation of a contraction in the irradiated wounds in
          comparison with the contralateral controls. Results obtained
          from 3 pairs of lesions are illustrated.

The first part of the biphasic response could be due to ultrasonically
stimulated shortening of contractile cells already present at the
wound site, possibly in response to changes in intracellular calcium
ion concentration[6]. The second stimulation occurred at a time when
myofibroblasts were already prominent components of the granulation
tissue which had developed in the region of the wound. The finding
that this stimulation of contraction persisted for several days after
the last treatment with ultrasound suggests that ultrasonic therapy
had produced a long term beneficial change in the granulation tissue.
It is possible that fibroblast migration into the wound area had
been enhanced by treatment with ultrasound, an observation already
noted in vitro[6,7] but not yet investigated in vivo. An increase
in the local population of fibroblasts, cells with the potential for
differentiation into contractile myofibroblasts, might well be
expected to produce a second increase in wound contraction once such
differentiation had taken place. The second part of the biphasic
response noted may thus be a consequence of earlier treatment with
ultrasound.

It is thus apparent, as predicted, that ultrasonic therapy stimulates wound contraction. The biological and biophysical mechanisms underlying this stimulation await detailed investigation.

ACKNOWLEDGEMENTS

We wish to thank Miss Marina Morris for skilled technical assistance, Spembly Ltd., U.K. for donation of a cryosurgical probe, and the National Fund for Research into Crippling Diseases (also known as Action Research) for financial support of this project.

REFERENCES

1. D. Montandon, G. Gabbiani, G.B. Ryan and G. Majno, The contractile fibroblast, its relevance in plastic surgery, Plast. Reconstruct. Surg. 52:286-290 (1973).
2. A.B. Galitsky and S.L. Levina, Vascular origin of trophic ulcers and application of ultrasound as pre-operative treatment to plastic surgery, Arch. Chir. Plast. 6:271-278 (1964).
3. M. Dyson, C. Francks and J. Suckling, Stimulation of healing of varicose ulcers by ultrasound, Ultrasonics 14:232-236 (1976).
4. G.R. ter Haar, M. Dyson and D. Talbert, Ultrasonically induced contraction in mouse uterine smooth muscle, Ultrasonics 16: 275-276 (1978).
5. S. Aryan, R. Enriquez and T.J. Krizek, Wound contraction and fibrocontractive disorders, Arch. Surg. 113:1034-1046 (1978).
6. C.L. Mummery, The effect of ultrasound on fibroblasts in vitro, (Ph.D. Thesis, University of London).
7. C.L. Mummery and M. Dyson, Increase in fibroblast motility in vitro by therapeutic levels of ultrasound, Ultrasound Med. Biol. (accepted for publication).

THE INFLUENCE OF ULTRASOUND ON MATRIX-BOUND ENZYMES

P. Schmidt and E. Rosenfeld

Institute of Applied Biophysics
Martin-Luther-University
Halle-Wittenberg, German Democratic Republic

and

J. Fischer

Central Institute of Genetics and Culture Plants Research
Academy of Science
Gatersleben, German Democratic Republic

INTRODUCTION

Immobilized enzymes are enzymes which have been linked to insoluble carriers either by chemical or physical attachement or by some form of entrapment. As heterogeneous catalysts they differ in many respects from their soluble counterparts and they are of theoretical and practical interest for many reasons. With the application of ultrasound two aims are purposed:

(i)   The alteration of the carrier structure by the action of high power ultrasound, which is of technological importance, and

(ii)   the study of ultrasonic effects on the enzymatic reaction itself.

MATERIAL AND METHODS

The carrier material used was polystyrene which consists of small spheres of about 1 mm diameter (VE Chemiekombinat Bitterfeld). In contrast to the ideal pore structure in the interior of the sphere

159

the sphere surface is disturbed during the polymerization process.
In this region a relatively compact layer hinders the penetration of
the substrate solution. To remove this layer the polystyrene spheres
were sonicated in aqueous suspension (100 mg dry polystyrene in 10 ml
aqua dest.). The sonication took place in a laboratory disintegrator
at 22 KHz and 300 W/cm^2. The study of ultrasonic effects on the
enqymatic reaction itself was carried out at 10.65 MHz and approximately 200 mW/cm^2 in a stirred tank reactor. The enzyme and substrate
for the reaction kinetic investigations were α-amylase from Asp.
oryzae (NOVO A/S, Denmark) and starch (Merck, Darmstadt), respectively. The temperature of the stirred solution was kept constant at
37°C by means of a thermostat. The reaction was stopped by separating
the solution containing the substrate and the reaction product
(maltose), through a filter. Afterwards chemical analysis could be
carried out[1]. The protein binding experiments were conducted with
chymotrypsin (Spofa, Prague).

RESULTS AND DISCUSSION

Ultrasonic Effects on the Carrier Material

The erosive action of cavitational ultrasound alters the surface
properties of the carrier material. After 20 minutes sonication at
22 KHz and 300 W/cm^2 the outer sphere layer is completely removed
and the porous matrix material comes to the fore. This can be
demonstrated by means of scanning electron microscopy. These results
are published elsewhere[2]. The penetration depth of the sonic
action can be estimated by means of transmission electron microscopic
pictures (Fig. 1.). The matrix structure is changed within a range
of 20 μm from the surface.

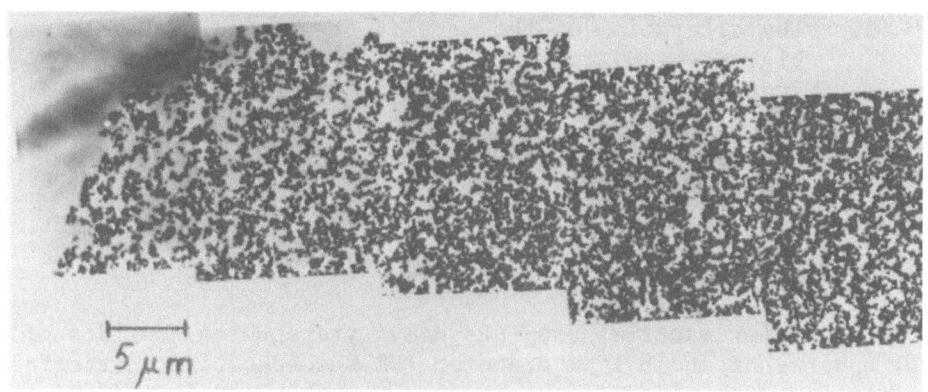

Fig. 1.   Transmission electron picture of the sonicated sample.

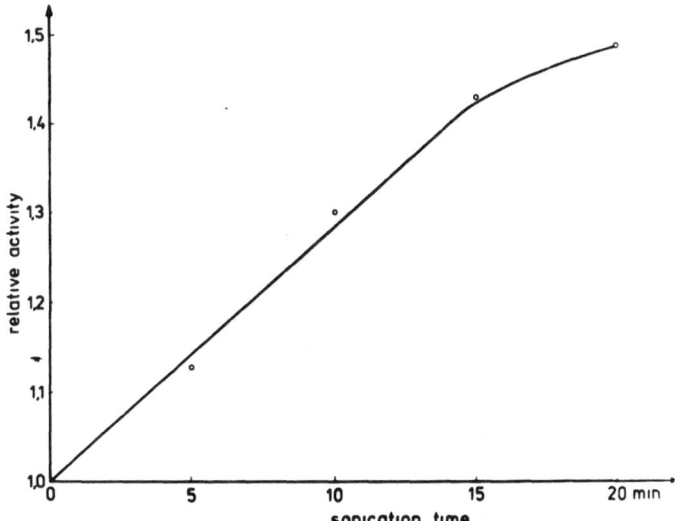

Fig. 2.   Increase of the activity of α-amylase in dependence on the
          sonicated time.

The sound-induced surface change of the polystyrene spheres is
accompanied by an increase in the activity of the enzyme-carrier
complex. In Fig. 2. the activity of immobilized α-amylase is plotted
versus the sonication time. The activity of the enzyme bond on a
20 minute sonicated carrier is increased by about 50% in relation
to the original material.

The biochemical characterization of the carrier properties was
accomplished by means of reaction kinetic measurements. The reaction
rate is described quantitatively by the Michaelis-Menten-Equation:

$$v = \frac{V_{max} \cdot S}{K_m + S}$$

v	reaction rate
V_{max}	maximum reaction rate
S	substrate concentration
K_m	Michaelis constant

A decrease in the Michaelis constant can be interpreted as an
intensification of the transport process during the reaction.

Fig. 3. shows the Lineweaver-Burk-plot of the enzyme-carrier-
complex using the untreated and the sonicated material. The abszissa
intercept and the ordinate intercept give the K_m-value and the
theoretical maximum reaction rate, respectively. V_{max} is the same

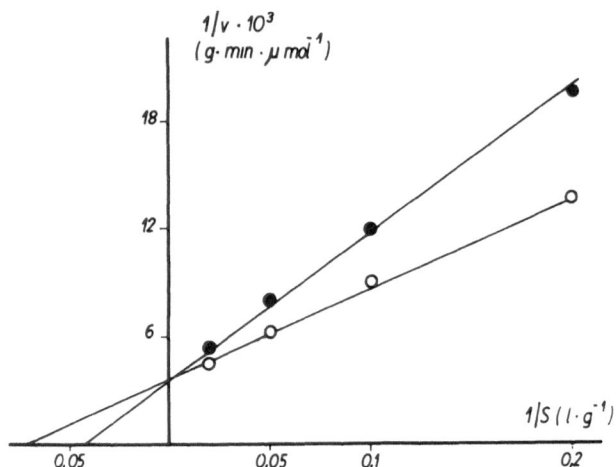

Fig. 3. Lineweaver-Burk-plot of the Michaelis-Menten-Equation.
o - sonicated sample; ● - unsonicated sample.

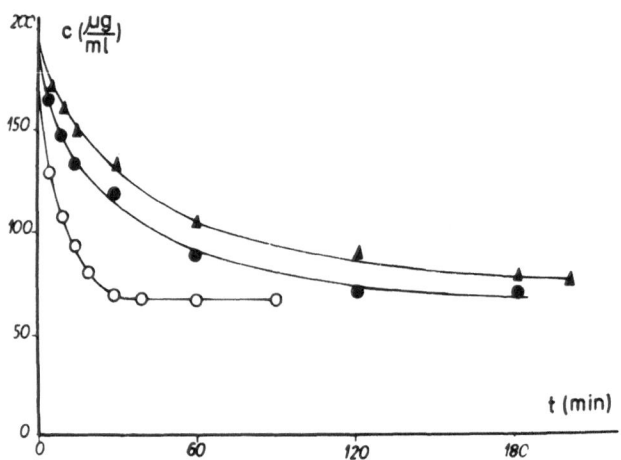

Fig. 4. Time dependence of adsorption of chymorypsin on
sonicated (o) and unsonicated (▲, ●) polystyrene.

in both cases (280 μmol/min.g). K_m amounts to 23.8 g/l and 13.7 g/l
for the untreated and sonicated carrier. The diffusion rate can also
be demonstrated by means of protein binding to the carrier matrix.
Fig. 4. represents the decrease in the concentration of chymotrypsin
in the solution due to protein binding to the matrix dependent on
the reaction time. The equilibrium is normally reached after 2 to
3 hours. In the sonicated sample, however, this process is complete
after 30 minutes.

Summarizing the first part of this investigation, one can
conclude that ultrasonic treatment of a polystyrene matrix can
positively influence the transport processes during the biochemical
heterogeneous catalysis.

The Influence of Ultrasound on the Enzymatic Reaction

The effect of high frequency ultrasound on the reaction rate
of immobilized α-amylase is demonstrated in Fig. 5. The diagram
shows the Lineweaver-Burk-plot of the Michaelis-Menten-Equation.
The slope of the curve of the sonicated sample is samller than that

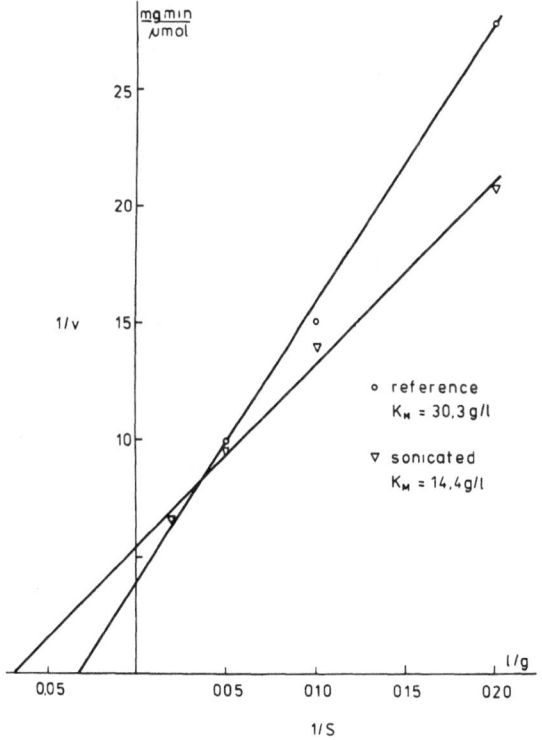

Fig. 5. Lineweaver-Burk-plot of the Michaelis-Menten-Equation of
the sonicated and unsonicated enzymatic reaction.

of the unsonicated one. The K_m-values are 14.4 g/1 and 30.3 g/1, respectively. The decrease in the K_m-value can be interpreted as an acceleration in the diffustion process in the vicinity of the immobilized enzyme molecules. There are several sonic effects which could explain such behavior.

1.   Rise in Temperature

The temperature rise can be caused by the absorption of the polystyrene sphere, adiabatic compression in the solution, and heating by viscous energy dissipation in a shell surrounding the sphere and heat conduction into the sphere. A rough calculation shows the temperature increase to be not higher than one degree, which cannot explain the increase in the reaction rate.

2.   Influence on Transport Mechanisms

Two types of diffusion processes play an important role during the enzymitic reaction[3,4]:

- film or exterior diffusion, and

- pore or internal diffusion.

To eliminate the first portion of the diffusion limitation the reactor is carefully stirred. However, an intensification of the liquid exchange near the surface of the sphere, due to acoustic streaming movements, cannot be excluded. The internal diffusion will be greatly dependent on the radius of the carrier ducts as well as on the sound frequency. At 10 MHz the acoustic boundary layer thickness is about 1800 Å[5]. Since the mean pore radius is approximately 700 Å, microstreaming would seem unlikely. However, in some cases the so-called invasion pores can reach a radius of some micrones. In these large capillaries an additional flow into the carrier body is conceivable.

In all cases discussed here the carrier material particles are assumed to behave as ridged balls. If elastic deformations are taken into consideration, resonance phenomena could contribute significantly to the transport processes.

REFERENCES

1.   P. Bernfeld, Methods Enzymol. 1_145 (1955).
2.   E. Rosenfeld, P. Schmidt and J. Fischer, in "Proceed. UBIOMED IV", Visegrad (1979).
3.   L. Goldstein, Methods Enzymol. 44:397 (1976).
4.   J-M. Engasser, Biochim. Biophys. Acta 526_301 (1978).

5.   M.E. Arkhangel'skii and Yu.G. Statnikov, Diffusion in hetero-
     geneous systems, in "Physical Principles of Ultrasonic
     Technology, Vol. $\overline{2^{\pi}}$, L.D. Rozenberg, ed., Plenum Press,
     New York, London (1973).

ELECTROKINETIC PROPERTIES OF ISOLATED CELLS EXPOSED TO LOW LEVELS OF ULTRASOUND

I. Hrazdira and J. Adler

Department of Biophysics, Faculty of Medicine
University J. E. Purkyne, Brno
Czechoslovakia

The rapid expansion of ultrasonic diagnostic procedures in many branches of medicine has increased the need for a better understanding of the basic biophysical events. Up to now the appreciation of possible hazards has been based mainly on the findings of chromosome aberrations of sonicated cells. Recently, however, it has been suggested that chromosome-breakages may not be the most sensitive indicator of cell damage, because certain biological reactions are affected even by ultrasonic intensities used in diagnostics. Detectable effects on DNA and growth patterns of animal cells at the temporal averaged spatial peak intensity of 45.5 $mWcm^{-2}$ were demonstrated by Liebeskind et al. (1979). Pizzarello et al. (1979) have shown that mouse lymphosarcoma exhibits reduced transplantability following exposure to an average acoustic output of 1.5 mW. Cellular attachment of cultured human cells has been found to be a sensitive indicator of the ultrasound effect at an output of 1.76 mW (Siegel et al. 1979). Miller et al. (1979) have found platelet aggregation induced by ultrasound at peak intensities of 16 - 32 $mWcm^{-2}$. All these findings show that ultrasound is able to produce alteration of a sensitive biological system even at intensities below 1 kWm^{-2}.

The cellular surface plays a significant role in a number of cell interactions with external factors. In our previous investigations, changes of the surface charge under the ultrasonic action at therapeutic intensities were proved (Hrazdira and Adler, 1980). In the present paper the influence of low intensity ultrasound on surface properties of human erythrocytes was investigated. Washed erythrocytes of fresh human citrated blood suspended in phosphate buffer at pH 7.4 or in isotonic sucrose were subjected to ultrasonic action at diagnostic exposure levels. A laboratory generator with two nonfocused transducers 20 mm in diameter (frequency 2 MHz and

6 MHz) was used as the source of ultrasonic pulses (pulse width $2\mu/s$, repetition frequency 2 kHz). The instantaneous temporal peak–spatial peak intensity was 6.4 kWm^{-2}, the temporal average–spatial average intensity was estimated at 26 Wm^{-2}. Samples of 20% erythrocyte suspension in amounts of 5 ml were sonicated in a vertical ultrasonic field for 30 minutes at 20°C. Immediately after ultrasonic treatment the electrokinetic properties of erythrocytes and their agglutination ability were determined.

The electrophoretic mobility (EPM) was measured in a horizontal electrophoretic chamber.

The results have shown a statistically significant increase of the EPM (Table 1.).

Table 1.   EPM of human erythrocytes treated by
           diagnostic ultrasound.

Specimen	Time interval between treatment and measurement	
	10 minutes	120 minutes
Control	11.95 ± 0.45	11.91 ± 0.43
2 MHz	14.54 ± 0.71	12.38 ± 0.56
6 MHz	15.56 ± 0.42	11.71 ± 0.47

EPM in Tiselius units (10^{-7} $ms^{-1}v^{-1}cm$)

The EPM of erythrocytes treated at 2 MHz frequency increased by 21%. The frequency of 6 MHz was more effective producing an average increase of 30%.

In parallel experiments the aggregation ability of erythrocytes induced by polyethylene glycol was established microscopically. The aggregation ability of sonicated erythrocytes was decreased and showed a shift to higher concentration of polyethylene glycol solutions. Also in these experiments the frequency of 6 MHz was more effective producing a statistically significant decrease by 15.4% the frequency of 2 MHz has produced an insignificant decrease by 6.2% only.

Both findings give evidence for an increase of the electrokinetic potential of sonicated cells due to transient alterations of the spatial distribution of ions in the electrical bilayer on the cell surface. As the efficacious mechanism the mechanical stress involving microstreaming and mocroshearing has been suggested. For the different efficacy of both frequencies used, however, no satisfactory explanation has been found to date.

SUMMARY

The influence of 2 MHz and 6 MHz ultrasound at diagnostic intensity level on surface electric properties of human erythrocytes has been investigated by means of cell electrophoresis and aggregation ability measurements. It has been demonstrated a transient increase of electrophoretic mobility by 21% and 30% at 2 MHz and 6 MHz respectively and a reduction of aggregation ability in polyethylene glycol solutions by 6.2% and 15.4% at the same frequencies. Both findings have been related to the ultrasonically induced increase in the electrokinetic potential of erythrocytes.

REFERENCES

Adler, J., and Hrazdira, I., 1980, Scripta Medica Fac. Med. Univ. Brun Purk., 53,6:329-332.

Liebeskind, D., Bases, R., Elequin, F., Neubort, S., Leifer, R., Goldberg, R., and Koenigsberg, M., 1979, Radiology, 131:179-184.

Miller, D. L., Nyborg, W. L., and Whitcomb, C. C., 1979, Science, 205:505-507.

Pizzarello, D. J., Vivino, A., and Newall, J., 1978, Exp. Cell. Biol., 46:240-245.

Siegel, E., Goddard, J., James, A. E. Jr., and Siegel, E. P., 1979, Radiology, 133:175-179.

INTERACTIONS OF ULTRASOUND WITH PLATELETS

AND THE BLOOD COAGULATION SYSTEM

A.R. Williams

Department of Medical Biophysics
University of Manchester, Medical School
Manchester M13 9PT, England, U.K.

The recalcification time of whole blood is a measure of the time taken to form strands of fibrin in vitro after the addition of enough calcium ions to overcome the effect of the anticoagulant. This time was significantly shortened (i.e. the blood sample rendered more clottable) after the samples had been exposed to continuous wave 1 MHz ultrasound at space averaged intensities within the range 0.065 to 2 W/cm^2[1]. The blood samples (each 1.5 ml) were contained within a siliconized Pyrex[R] glass tube (1.1 cm i.d. and 1.5 cm long) attached centrally at 90° to a hollow glass stem so that it resembled the letter "T". The open ends of the glass tube were covered with an acoustically transparent window of cling film held in position by means of rubber O-rings. This sample chamber was mounted in a 37°C water bath on axis with and in the near field of the transducer. The formation of standing waves was minimized by the incorporation of a highly absorbing bath of castor oil at the far end of the exposure tank.

Electron micrographic investigations were performed on the thrombi produced by the recalcification of human platelet rich plasma (PRP; i.e. anticoagulated whole blood with the erythrocytes and most of the white cells removed by centrifugation). Platelet thrombi from irradiated samples contained some debris from disrupted platelets and the remaining intact platelets were abnormal in that (a) they were more vacuolated, (b) they formed a larger number of smaller aggregates, and (c) their clot retraction mechanism was impaired[2]. These abnormalities could be duplicated by incubating normal platelet debris from homogenized platelet suspensions[2].

A suspension of PRP is turbid because the larger number of
individual small platelets scatter the incident light. However, if
the platelets are stimulated to undergo their normal physiological
function, or are subjected to an adverse physical or chemical
environment, they adhere to each other until they form a smaller
number of large aggregates which permit more light to pass through
the sample. The rate of change of light transmission during
aggregation can be measured (i.e. platelet aggregometry) and is an
extremely sensitive technique to evaluate platelet function in vitro.
The apparatus described above was modified by passing a light beam
through the stirred platelet suspension at right angles to the axis
of the ultrasound beam. It was found that under certain conditions
ultrasonic irradiation alone could initiate aggregation of human
platelets, and that the traces obtained (e.g. Fig. 1.), were virtually
identical to those produced by adding different amounts of Adenosine
Diphosphate (ADP), the normal physiological initiator of platelet
aggregation.

Fig. 1. shows that at a constant space averaged intensity of
1.8 W/cm^2 (continuous wave) the extent of ultrasound induced aggregation decreased as the frequency was increased from 0.75 to 3 MHz[3].
This observation, together with the electron micrographic results
outlined above, strongly indicates that some form of cavitational
activity may be disrupting some of the platelets.

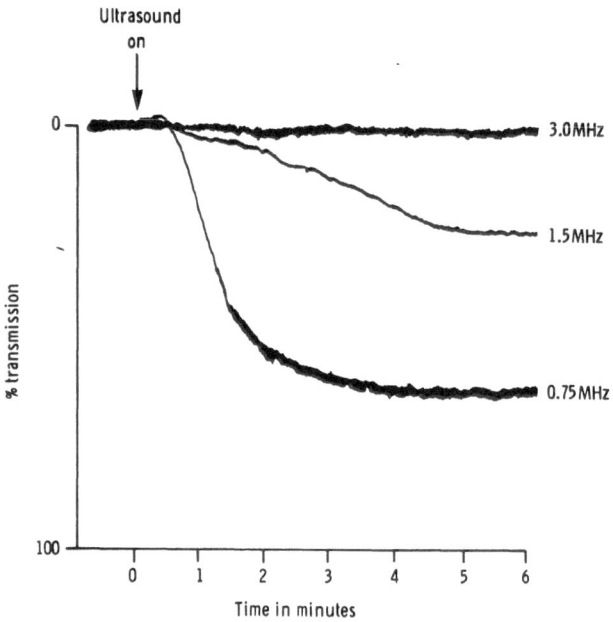

Fig. 1.   Platelet aggregation induced by 1.8 W/cm^2 of ultrasound
          at different frequencies.

For any one human donor the amount of aggregation produced by any given ultrasonic exposure at 0.75 MHz was remarkably constant. However, PRP from different donors sometimes exhibited wide variation (Fig. 2.). It is known that PRP from different donors may have a different sensitivity to aggregation by ADP and so in a separate series of experiments aliquots of PRP from the same donors used to compile Fig. 2. were exposed to near threshold levels of 4 µM and 10 µM ADP. The number on each curve in Fig. 2. refers to the sensitivities of those platelets to ADP-induced aggregation with number (1) being the most sensitive and number (5) being the least sensitive. It can be seen that the most sensitive platelets required a lower ultrasonic intensity to induce aggregation, and that the maximal extent of this aggregation was always greater than that obtained with less sensitive platelets[3].

Thus, the "threshold" intensities observed for the induction of platelet aggregation (Fig. 3.) appear to reflect the concentration of an aggregating agent (possibly ADP itself released from damaged or disrupted platelets), which has to be attained within that medium. This hypothesis is supported by the observation that PRP samples irradiated at intensities less than the "threshold" necessary to induce aggregation were refractory when challenged with more ADP[3].

β-Thromboglubulin (β-TG) is a protein found only within human platelets which is liberated when the platelets are disrupted or undergo their normal physiological release reaction[4]. Its concentration can be measured with an accuracy of about 2 to 3 ng/ml by means of a specific radioimmunoassay and normal plasma values range

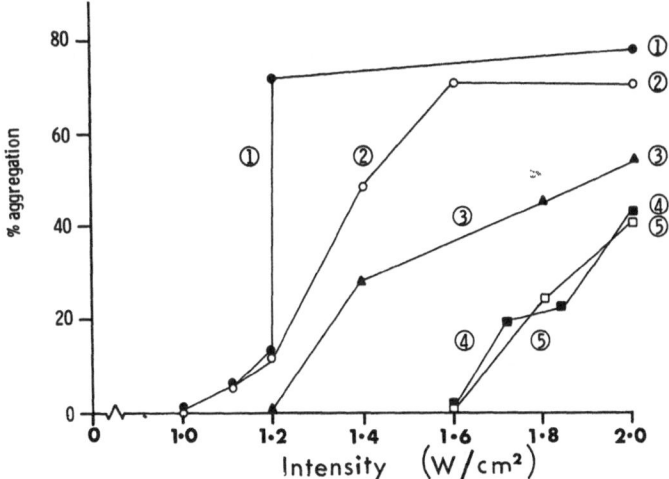

Fig. 2. Ultrasound-induced aggregation of PRP from different human donors irradiated at 0.75 MHz.

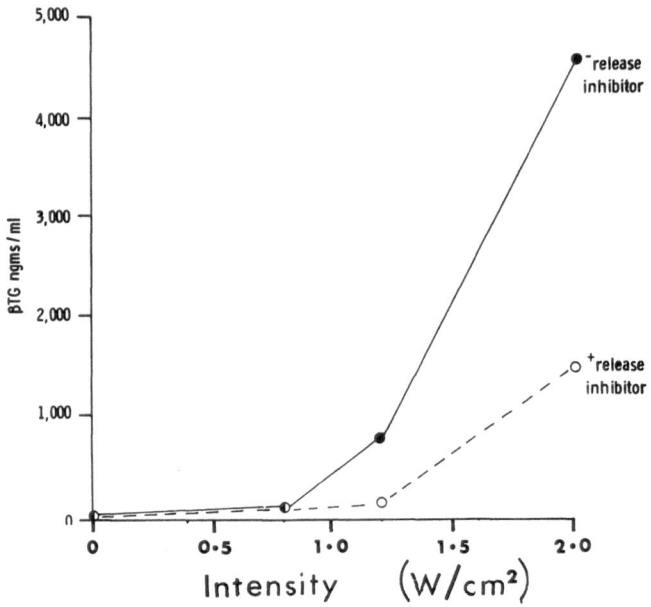

Fig. 3. Release of β-Thromboglobulin from human platelets
at 0.75 MHz.

from 20 to 40 ng/ml rising to more than 5.000 ng/ml in serum where
all the platelets have released.

The uppermost curve in Fig. 3. (- release inhibitor) shows the
additional amount of β-TG released into the plasma when anticoagulated whole blood was arradiated at 0.75 MHz. This shows that
abouve about 0.8 W/cm^2 there was a steep intensity-dependent
increase in the amount of β-TG released into the plasma[5]. There
was no sharp cut-off or "threshold" as the ultrasonic intensity was
reduced below 0.8 W/cm^2. Other (unreported) measurements showed
that the curve of β-TG release began to merge with the baseline at
intensities below about 0.6 W/cm^2, but the precise value varied from
day to day.

The lower curve in Fig. 3. (+ release inhibitor) was obtained
using the same blood sample as the upper trace except that it
contained a mixture of EDTA and theophylline which prevented the
platelets undergoing their normal release reaction. It can be seen
that this inhibitor decreased the amount of β-TG released by ultrasound to about 30% of the control value. The only plausible
mechanism for liberating β-TG from these functionally-inert platelets
is by disrupting them. This argument in favor of cavitation is
supported by the fact that high levels of β-TG release were always
accompanied by a corresponding increase in the levels of plasma
haemoglobin from disrupted erythocytes[5].

All of the above results indicate that some form of cavitational activity is being generated at "suprathreshold" intensities of ultrasound which subsequently disrupts a small proportion of the platelet and (if they are also present) erythrocyte populations. When enough cells have been disrupted, materials (including ADP) liberated from these disrupted cells will induce other intact functional platelets to undergo their release reaction (liberating β-TG and more ADP) and to aggregate.

The "threshold" intensity for any one of the effects reported above is increased if the sample to be irradiated is degassed or not stirred during the sonication procudure. Conversely, the "threshold" intensity is decreased if the samples to be irradiated are bubbled, agitated, stirred or aerated. The lowest "threshold" values obtainable in vitro are found when microscopic gas bodies are deliberately introduced into the sonication medium. These micron-sized gas bubbles tend to dissolve spontaneously, but they may be stabilized within the uniformly sized pores of hydrophobic Nuclepore[R] membranes. When these stable gas bubbles are present, human platelets can be disrupted at average intensities as low as 8 mW/cm^2 at 1.6 MHz (A.R. Williams and D.L. Miller, unpublished observations) and can be induced to aggregate by the ultrasonic field emitted by a conventional doppler diagnostic instrument[6].

It is therefore extremely difficult to extrapolate from these in vitro measurements to the in vivo situation. Blood within the body must contain gaseous nucleation sites because these are the starting points from which gas bubbles grow during decompression. However, these cannot be studied in vitro because there is no practicable way of removing blood from an animal without exposing it to foreigh surfaces or otherwise changing its content of nucleation sites by adding foreign substances such as anticoagulants. Dr B.V. Chater and I therefore attempted to duplicate some of the experiments described above to see whether we could produce similar effects in vivo.

An antecubital vein in one arm of healthy adult human volunteers was cannulated and sequential 2.5 ml samples of blood were collected in plastic tubes containing EDTA and theophylline as anticoagulant and inhibitor of the platelet release reaction. Immediately after the first sample (Control 1) had been collected the stationary 0.75 MHz transducer over the upstream portion of the vein was activated at the highest intensity which that volunteer would tolerate (0.25 to 0.34 W/cm^2, continuous wave). After the test sample had been collected the transducer was switched off and the next one or two ml of blood to emerge from the catheter was discarded before collecting a second control sample. It was found that there was no significant elevation of β-TG levels in the test samples[7].

One criticism of this in vivo series is that the intensities used were too low to demonstrate a positive effect. An animal model was therefore developed whereby similar sequential samples could be withdrawn from the inferior vena cava of anaesthetized rabbits before during, and after irradiation at 0175 MHz[8]. Rabbit platelets do not contain β-TG but they are loaded with Histamine which is released under similar conditions. Histamine was released within the intact blood vessels in vivo when the blood was forced to cavitate by the application of 25 KHz probe to the outside of the vessel wall. However, spatially averaged intensities of up to 10 W/cm² at 0.75 MHz for 30 to 40 seconds did not result in the release of detectable quantities of Histamine from the platelets or of haemoglobin from erythocytes in vivo[8].

Contradictory results were obtained by Wong and Watmough[9] who found that 0.75 MHz ultrasound directed into the beating hearts of anaesthetized mice through their diaphragm resulted in the lysis of erythrocytes (and presumably also platelets). It is highly probable that the turbulence and large pressure changes occurring within the beating heart enhanced the nucleation characteristics of the blood and so lowered the "threshold" intensity for generating ultrasonic cavitation in vivo.

CONCLUSIONS

1.   Ultrasonic cavitation appears to be the primary mechanism causing damage to platelets in vitro.

2.   Most in vitro experimental arrangements will increase the probability of generating cavitation.

3.   Platelet damage dows not apparently occur in vivo at therapeutic frequencies and intensities if one irradiates quiescent or orderly flowing blood.

4.   It is not advisable to subject turbulent blood flow or blood containing undissolved gas bubbles to ultrasonic irradiation.

REFERENCES

1.   A.R. Williams, W.D. O'Brien, Jr. and B.S. Coller, Exposure to ultrasound decreases the recalcification time of platelet rich plasma, Ultrasound in Med. & Biol. 2:311 (1976).
2.   A.R. Williams, S.M. Sykes and W.D. O'Brien, Jr., Ultrasonic exposure modifies platelet morphology and function in vitro, Ultrasound in Med. & Biol. 2:311 (1976).

3.   B.V. Chater and A.R. Williams, Platelet aggregation induced in
     vitro by therapeutic ultrasound, Thrombosis and Haemostasis
     3:640 (1977).
4.   C.A. Ludlam, S. Moore, A.E. Bolton, D.S. Pepper and J.D. Cash,
     The release of human platelet-specific protein measured by
     a radioimmunoassay, Thrombosis Res. 6:543 (1975).
5.   A.R. Williams, B.V. Chater, K.A. Allen, M.R. Sherwood and
     J.H. Sanderson, Release of β-Thromboglobulin from human
     platelets by therapeutic intensities of ultrasound, Brit. J.
     Haematol. 40:123 (1978).
6.   D.L. Miller, W.L. Nyborg and C.C. Whitcomb, Platelet aggregation
     induced by ultrasound under specialised conditions in vitro,
     Science 3:505 (1979).
7.   A.R. Williams, B.V. Chater, K.A. Allen and J.H. Sanderson, The
     use of β-Thromoglobulin to detect platelet damage by thera-
     peutic ultrasound in vivo, J. Clin. Ultrasound (1981) in
     Press.
8.   A.R. Williams and B.V. Chater, Absence of detectable thrombo-
     genic hazard associated with the the exposure of non-turbulent
     blood to therapeutic ultrasound in vivo, Article in
     preparation.
9.   Y.S. Wong and D.J. Watmough, Haemolysis of red blood cells in
     vitro and in vivo caused by therapeutic ultrasound at
     0.75 MHz, Paper C 14 at the Ultrasound Interaction in Biology
     and Medicine Symposium, Reinhardsbrunn, East Germany,
     No. 10-14 (1980).

HAEMOLYSIS OF RED BLOOD CELLS IN VITRO AND IN VIVO INDUCED BY

ULTRASOUND AT 0.75 MHz AND AT THERAPEUTIC INTENSITY LEVELS

Y.S. Wong and D.J. Watmough

Department of Bio-Medical Physics and Bio-Engineering
University of Aberdeen, Fosterhill
Aberdeen, Scotland

INTRODUCTION

The physical mechanisms by which ultrasound can modify or damage biological materials has been comprehensively discussed by Nyborg[1]. These include microstreaming, thermal effects and a range of cavitation type phenomena. It is well known that an acoustically excited bubble can cause haemolysis of red cells[2]. The shearing stresses on the red cells caused by associated microstreaming is sufficient to damage cell membranes. Release of haemoglobin causes changes in optical absorbance when the treated samples are subsequently measured by spectrophotometry. Nyborg[1] and others have remarked that there is little information on cavitation in bulk animal tissues which are characteristically opaque. The objective of the work described here was to direct ultrasound from an unmodified therapeutic generator (Sonacel, Rank Stanley, Cox, Ware, Hertfordshire, England) at the hearts of small animals in an attempt to detect or exclude haemolysis in vivo. The need for this investigation arises from the now wide-spread use of ultrasound as a therapeutic agent to treat a variety of conditions[3]. Furthermore, there is considerable interest in the possibility of treating malignant tumors with focussed or over-lapping ultrasound fields[4] with a view to producing local hyperthermia. Clearly it is vital to know if there are likely to be any untoward side-effects arising from such treatment.

EXPERIMENTAL

(a) Sonication of Human Erythrocytes In Vitro

     Peripheral venous blood was drawn from the right antecubital
vein of one of us (S.Y.W.) under full aseptic and gentle conditions
to prevent any unnecessary or excessive stresses to the erythrocytes
by syringes and needles. Blood was collected in tubes containing
potassium ethylene diamine tetra-acetate to prevent clotting by
gentle mixing. 20 ml 0.9% sodium chloride solution was used to dilute
2 ml of the sequestrene blood, then collected in a 25 ml beaker with
gentle mixing at all times. Each such specimen was insonated for

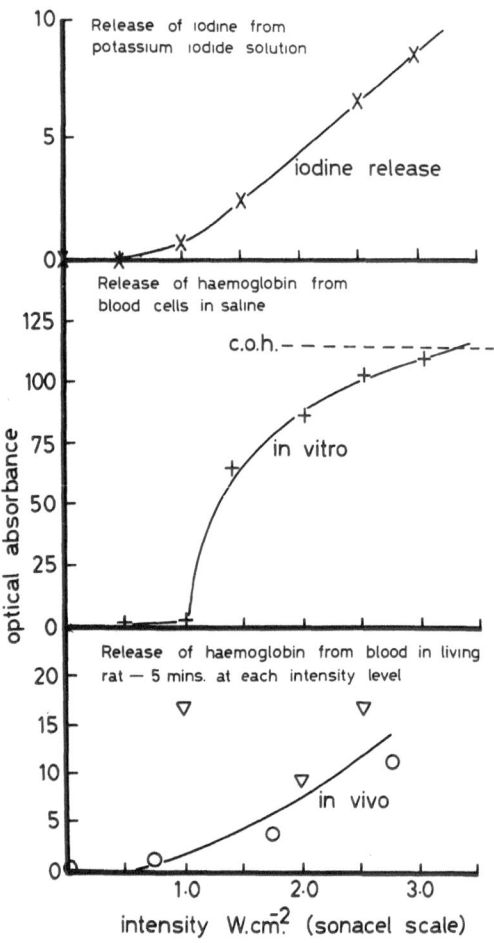

Fig. 1. (upper curve) test for cavitation using potassium iodide
         solution; (middle curve) haemolysis of human red blood cells
         in normal saline; (lower curve) effect of 5 min. treatments
         with 0.75 MHz ultrasound on blood using intact rats.

5 minutes at particular intensity levels with the transducer just
below the liquid surface. The system gave rise to a standing wave
field which we did not attempt to minimise since it represents a
similar situation to that which occurs at bone-tissue interfaces
within the body. The controls comprised, (a) normal blood,
(b) 1:10 diluted normal blood, (c) 1 in 10 normal blood at 45°C for
10 minutes (to exclude thermal effects as a mechanism of damage),
and (d) 1:10 diluted normal blood, using distilled water instead of
normal saline to five a curve for complete osmotic haemolysis. The
samples and controls were quantified using an u-v spectrophotometer
(Unicam SP800) in order to assess the degree of haemolysis.
Absorbance data versus nominal intensity levels (W/cm^{-2}) are shown
in the middle curve of Fig. 1. Separate experiments using a radiation
force balance were made to estimate the corresponding spation average
intensities and these are shown in Fig. 2. The spatial peak intensity
was estimated using the Kossoff approximation[5] as being about five
times the spatial average, though this data refers to the profile
of the beam in progressive form. The energy density is further
enhanced by reflection from the base of the sonication vessel.

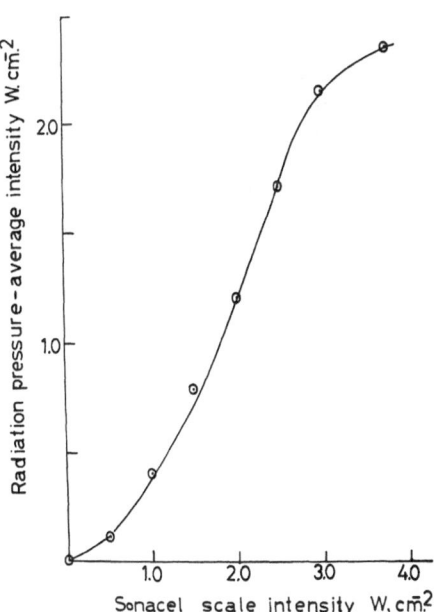

Fig. 2. Relation between scale values of intensity of Sonacel
         generator and measurements made using a radiation balance
         to determine average values. The ultrasound was continuous
         wave and the spatial peak values were estimated to be about
         five times the average values.

Increase in intensity leads to a fairly sharp onset of haemolysis at 0.5 W/cm^{-2} (spatial average) increasing to almost complete haemolysis at 2.0 W/cm^{-2} (spatial average). Microstreaming around sonically induced bubbles could be seen in the treatment vessel and is assumed to be responsible for the observed effect at 0.75 MHz. The optical absorbance was measured at 414 nm -- because it gives the largest variation with sound intensity.

(b) Study of Cavitation Using Potassium Iodide Solution

Iodine release from potassium iodide solution with added carbon tetrachloride is used as a test[6] for the presence of cavitation. Solutions containing 0.5 g KI together with 5 ml CCl$_4$ and 25 ml distilled water were made up and treated with ultrasound from the Sonacel transducer. At each intensity level, 5 minute treatments were given and varying amounts of iodine were released. The effect was quantified by the optical absorbance of the iodine using the Unicam SP800 u-v spectrophotometer. A threshold for iodine release of about 0.5 W/cm^{-2} (spatial average) was found; thereafter the absorbance increased steadily with increasing intensity. The absorption at 350 nm was used for comparison of the samples.

(c) Experimental

A series of rats were each anaesthetized under ether in a bell jar and then laid supine on an operating table. The area below the rib cage was shaved and so was an area over the aortic arch. The animals were maintained under anaesthesia by intermittently applying a gauze soaked in ether to their mouth. The 0.75 MHz transducer was applied with coupling gel to the skin below the ribs and directed at the heart. Five minute treatments at a single (but different) intensity level was given to each animal. At the end of the treatment

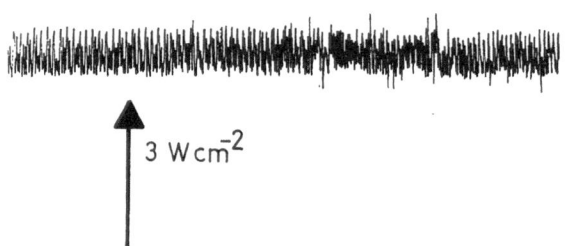

Fig. 3. Doppler trace of blood flow in aortic arch of a rat while being treated with ultrasound.

5 ml of blood was taken from the heart and subsequently analyzed as described in (a)*. Here also we found an intensity threshold of ~ 0.5 W/cm^{-2} (spatial average) for the onset of haemolysis and at higher intensity levels the degree of haemolysis increased. There were technical difficulties in trying to ensure that the transducer-skin coupling was comparable between different experiments and we could not even be sure that there was not time to time variation during a particular treatment.

A Doppler transducer (BV381) was placed so as to monitor blood flow in the aortic arch before and during sonication. Large spikes on some of the traces were noted after switching on the therapeutic ultrasound. Fig. 3. shows one example of this phenomena. Further work to establish whether these spikes are due to acoustically induced microbubbles in the circulation are under way in our laboratory. This possibility of in vivo cavitation cannot be ruled out. Sonically generated bubbles have been observed previously[7] in the transparent tails of small tropical fish.

DISCUSSIONS AND CONCLUSIONS

At intensities above about 0.5 W/cm^{-2} (spatial average) cavitation type phenomena have been found to cause haemolysis of human red blood cells. The frequency was 0.75 MHz, the lowest used in ultrasound therapy and that most likely to cause cavitation type effects. There was a threshold below which haemolysis did not appear to occur, at least in 5 minute treatment times. Above the threshold haemolysis rose rapidly becoming almost complete at 2.0 W/cm^{-2} (spatial average). The presence of cavitation, above a threshold of ~ 0.5 W/cm^{-2} (spatial average) was confirmed by the potassium iodide reduction test.

Sonication of a number of rats at various intensity levels each for periods of 5 minutes appears to show that sonication causes haemolysis in vivo. There is probably a similar threshold in this case as well. Increasing the intensity at fixed treatment times increases the degree of haemolysis observed. Doppler traces of blood flow in the aortic arch suggest that microbubbles may be induced within the circulation of intact animals by therapeutic levels of ultrasound but further work to clarify this is under way. The potential use of ultrasound to produce local hyperthermia in tumors makes more urgent the need to understand and control effects such as those described in this paper.

---

*The animals were all sacrificed without recovery from the anaesthetic.

SUMMARY

Human red blood cells suspended in normal saline were haemolyzed by therapeutic ultrasound of intensity $\sim$ 0.5 W/cm^{-2} (spatial average) and frequency 0.75 MHz. Such a threshold was shown to be due to a form of cavitation capable of reducing potassium iodide to free iodine in the presence of carbon tetrachloride. Application of therapeutic ultrasound to the hearts of intact living rats also produced haemolysis of red blood cells, the degree of haemolysis increasing with increasing intensity.

ACKNOWLEDGEMENT

This work has been generously supported by the Cancer Research Campaign.

REFERENCES

1. W.L. Nyborg, Physical mechanisms for biological effects of ultrasound, HEW publication (FDA) 78-8062 (1978).
2. J.A. Rooney, Haemolysis near an ultrasonically pulsating gas bubble, Sicence 169:869-871 (1970).
3. J.F. Lehmann and A.W. Guy, Ultrasound therapy, in "Interaction of Ultrasound and Biological Tissues", J.M. Reid and M.R. Sikov, eds., DHEW publication (FDA) 73-8008 (1972), pp. 141-152.
4. G.M. Hahn and D. Pounds, Heat treatment of solid tumors: why and how, Applied Radiol. Sept./Oct. 131-144 (1976).
5. G. Kossoff, The measurement of peak acoustic intensity generated by pulsed ultrasonic equipment, Ultrasonics 7:249-251 (1969).
6. A. Weissler, H.W. Cooper and S. Snyder, Chemical effects of ultrasonic waves; oxidation of potassium iodide solution by carbon tetrachloride, J. Am. Chem. Soc. 72:1769-1775 (1950).
7. D.J. Watmough, B. Pratt, M. Mallard and J.R. Mallard, The Biophysical effects of therapeutic ultrasound in vivo, V International Conference on Meidcal Physics, Jerusalem, Israel (1979).

ESR-SPECTROSCOPIC EXAMINATIONS OF ULTRASONICATED BLOOD

R. Glöckner and B. Milsch*

Institute of Pathology, Hospital-Centre
GDR 1242 Bad Saarow, PF 65 953

*Section of Physics, Karl-Marx-University
GDR 7010 Leipzig, Linnestrasse 5

In connection with examinations of the disruption of formed blood constituents ultrasound was applied to the disintegration – starting with investigations on ultrasonic hemolysis. We used a 20 KHz tube swinger with a power factor of 300 W/cm^2, that was developed by the Institute of Applied Biophysics at the University of Halle. When whole blood was sounded by a power factor of 200 W/cm^2 a complete destruction of cellular elements resulted within a period of 15 seconds, as was shown by an examination through a microscope. It was of interest whether detectable changes in the molecular region were induced by the sounding.

The electron-spin-resonance (ESR) spectroscopy is able to demonstrate paramagnetic centers in the biologic material[1,2]. Besides, the method allows one to make statements on the molecular changes in the region of these paramagnetic centers.

The ESR spectroscopy seemed to be capable of registering the changes produced in the molecular region by ultrasound immediately.

MATERIAL AND METHOD

Whole blood from clinically healthy people of both sexes that was made uncoagulable by sodiumcitrat was sounded with a 20 KHz tune swinger for different durations with changing intensity. After that the blood was dried at a temperature of 35°C and then placed in standard ESR quartz cuvettes. Untreated control samples of the same people were processed in the same way. The ESR instrument used

185

in this study was a Varian E 12 spectrometer equipped with the Varian
4540 temperature control unit.   In addition, for the low temperature
measurements a helium continuous flow cryostat ESR 9 (produced by
Oxford Instruments) was available.   This instrument secures the full
spectrometer sensitivity at low temperature needed for measurements
of biological samples.   Measurements were made at the three
temperatures (T=300, 123 and 4 K).   After careful positioning of the
sample tube in the ESR microwave cavity the samples were quickly
cooled down with a cooling rate of about 100 K/min.   In this way
our cooling procedure resembles a standard rapid freezing technique.

RESULTS AND DISCUSSION

Fig. 1. shows the ESR spectra obtained for an untreated blood
sample at T=300, 123 and 4 K.

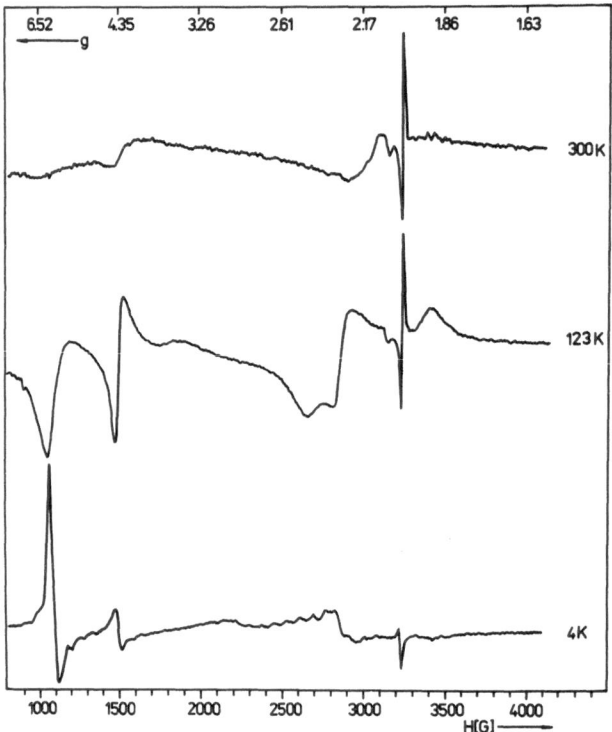

Fig. 1.   ESR spectra of an unsonicated whole blood sample at
           T=300, 123 and 4 K.   X-Band, modulation frequency 100 KHz,
           modulation amplitude 8 G, microwave power 5 mW for the
           300 and 123 K records, 0.1 mW for the 4 K record.   The
           gain was $6.3 \cdot 10^3$, $4 \cdot 10^3$, and $6.3 \cdot 10^2$ respectively.

It is clearly seen that ESR transitions with g-factors of
6.0, 4.3, 2.28, 2.0042, and 1.952 are well-resolved and the best
resolution is obtained at the lowest temperature T=4 K.

We interpret these line positions as follows. The ESR
experiment "sees" the immediate neighborhood of the iron ion in the
haem plane of the haemoglobin molecule in its different valency states
and "feels" the strength and the symmetry of the chemical binding to
the various ligand groups. The observed lines at $g_{||}$=2.0 and $g_{\perp}$=6.0
are due to the high spin ferric ion Fe^{3+} bound in the center of the
haemoglobin molecule. This ion feels a strong axial molecular field
directed normal to the haem plane and is bound mainly ionically. The
transition near g=4.3 can be explained in terms of high spin Fe^{3+}
ions placed in a site with a large component of rhombic molecular
field. The three different components g_x, g_y, and g_z are not resolved
in this experiment. Usually this signal is assigned to nonhaem iron
in proteins. The resonance with g=2.3 is typical for low spin iron
in protein. The ferric iron ion is strongly bound to the ligand and
possesses only one unpaired spin in the 3 d orbital, thus resulting
in a spin of S=1/2. At g=1.95 we found a resonance line often
obtained for iron in various biological samples, usually assigned to
an iron ion bound to the macromolecular structure of the protein
itself at a site with partial orthorhombic symmetry. Again in our
case g_x, g_y, and g_z are not resolved.

The ESR experiment detects free radicals in the sample. The
strong resonance at g=2.0042 with a line width of only 10 G is
observed at room temperature. G-factor, line width, and the
saturation behavior at room temperature point out that this resonance
is due to free radical species. It is partly overlapped by the
$g_{||}$=2.0 resonance of Fe^{3+}.

There are reports on ESR detection of Cu^{2+} in coerulopiasmin
($g_{||}$=2.209, $g_{\perp}$=2.056) in frozen human whole blood samples (Kawasaki
[3,4]. We were not able to obtain these resonances and put this
fact down to differing preparation methods.

Fig. 2. shows the ESR spectrum of sonicated blood samples. The
results give the same picture. There are no essential changes in the
position of the lines, in the width of the lines, and in the
intensities.

Resulting from what we have previously stated, it must be said
that a sounding with a frequency of 20 KHz with intensities of
10-200 W/cm^2 and a sounding duration of 30 seconds to 5 minutes in
steps of 30 seconds does not produce any changes in the spectrum.

Neither the existing paramagnetic centers changed nor do new
long-lived free radicals arise.

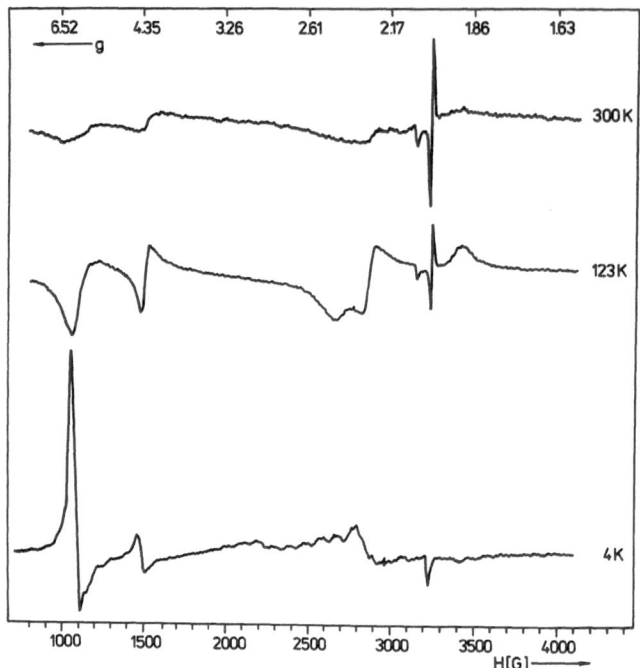

Fig. 2.   ESR spectra of an ultrasonicated whole blood sample at
          T=300, 123, and 4 K.   Spectrometer setting as above.

CONCLUSION

     As the method of detectable changes is a consequence of partly
profound changes in the molecular structure we come to the conclusion
that with regard to the given experimental conditions the mechanic
destruction of corpuscular elements with all its consequences is total
in this case.

SUMMARY

1.   Sonicated and unsonicated samples of human whole blood have been
     examined by the ESR spectroscopy.

2.   The sounding produced no changes in the spectrum, regardless of
     the period of sounding or its intensity.

3.   The obtained resonance lines are in agreement with the values
     given in the literature.

REFERENCES

1. H. M. Swartz et al, "Biological Application of Electron Spin
   Resonance", Wiley Interscience, New York (1972).
2. D. J. E. Ingram, "Biological and Biochemical Application of
   Electron Spin Resonance", Adam Hilger Ltd, London (1969).
3. H. Kawasaki et al., Electron spin resonance spectra of the
   bloods in diseased conditions, Kurume Med. J. 25:273 (1978).
4. R. A. Horn et al., ESR studies on properties of ceruloplasmin
   and transferrin in blood from human subjects and cancer
   patients, Cancer 43:2392 (1979).

NONLINEAR PROPAGATION OF ULTRASOUND IN LIQUID MEDIA

F. Dunn, W.K. Law and L.A. Frizzell

Bioacoustics Research Laboratory
University of Illinois.
Urbana, Illinois 61801, U.S.A.

It is well known that acoustic phenomena are fundamentally non-linear, though a large class of acoustical phenomena can be dealt with by linearizing the equations of motion leading to acceptable and usable solutions[1,2]. This is, of course, very convenient as the nonlinear relations are extremely difficult to deal with. However, it is necessary on occasion to have more details of the propagation processes, e.g., for a more profound understanding of the phenomena, than can be obtained from the linear theories. Thus, a program has been initiated to examine this question and preliminary measurements give an indication of the degree of non-linearity of biological media.

The equation of motion or the wave equation for acoustic phenomena is obtained by invoking three constitutive equations, viz. an equation of continuity, a dynamical equation, and an equation of state of the medium in which the propagation is to take place. In Lagrangian coordinates, these are respectively:

$$\rho = \rho_o \left(1 + \frac{\partial \xi}{\partial x}\right)^{-1}, \quad \rho \ddot{\xi} = -\frac{\partial p}{\partial x}, \quad \text{and} \quad c^2 = \frac{\partial p}{\partial \rho} \tag{1}$$

Here, ρ and ρ_o are the disturbed and undistrubed density, respectively, ξ is the particle displacement of the medium, p is the sound pressure, and x is the Lagrangian coordinate. Combining these equations leads to:

$$\ddot{\xi} = c^2 / \left(1 + \frac{\partial \xi}{\partial x}\right)^2 \xi'' \;,$$

the equation of motion obtained without approximation. It is seen that if a Hooke's law relationship for the equation of state is employed, such that $\partial p/\partial\rho$ is constant, and if the displacement amplitude of the wave is sufficiently small such that $\partial\xi/\partial x \ll 1$, the ordinary lossless wave equation is obtained, viz. $\ddot{\xi} = c^2\xi''$.

Now consider the situation wherein the displacement amplitude is not negligible and the quation of state is more complex than the simple Hooke's law relationship. The second point can be accommodated by considering the equation of state to be expanded in a Taylor's series for the isentropic case such that:

$$p-p_0 = \left(\frac{\partial p}{\partial\rho}\right)_{S,\rho=\rho_0} (\rho-\rho_0) + \frac{1}{2!} \left(\frac{\partial^2 p}{\partial\rho^2}\right)_{S,\rho=\rho_0} (\rho-\rho_0)^2 +$$

$$+ \frac{1}{3!} \left(\frac{\partial^3 p}{\partial\rho^3}\right)_{S,\rho=\rho_0} (\rho-\rho_0)^3 + \ldots$$

It is convenient to rewrite this in series form

$$p-p_0 = As + \frac{B}{2!} s^2 + \frac{C}{3!} s^3 + \ldots ,$$

where $A = \rho_0 \left(\frac{\partial p}{\partial\rho}\right)_{S,\rho=\rho_0} = \rho_0 c_0^2 ;$

$$B = \rho_0^2 \left(\frac{\partial^2 p}{\partial\rho^2}\right)_{S,\rho=\rho_0} ;$$

$$C = \rho_0^3 \left(\frac{\partial^3 p}{\partial\rho^3}\right)_{S,\rho=\rho_0}$$

and $s = (\rho-\rho_0)/\rho_0$.

Thus the speed of sound becomes:

$$c^2 = c_0^2 \left[1 + \left(\frac{B}{A}\right) s + \left(\frac{B}{2A}\right) s^2 + \ldots\right]$$

and the equation of motion is, for the case where only the first
two terms in the series are retained,

$$\ddot{\xi} = \frac{c_o^2}{(1+\xi')^{2+B/A}} \xi'' .$$

Here it is seen that for the situation where the displacement amplitude cannot be neglected, the parameter B/A becomes a measure of
the nonlinearity of the propagating medium.

A consequence of the propagation described by this relation in
a fluid medium is that an originally sinusoidal, monochromatic wave
becomes distorted as it propagates, harmonics are generated, and the
amplitude of these harmonics is a function of the distance from the
source[3]. The harmonics have zero amplitude at the source, increase
to a maximum value at a position from the source at which the effect
of absorption processes balances such harmonic production and propagation occurs as under linear conditions well beyond this point.

The quantity B/A can be approximated as:

$$\frac{B}{A} = \frac{2\rho_o c_o^3}{\pi f} \left[\frac{p_2 (x)}{x p_1^2 (o)}\right] \Bigg|_{x p_1 (o) \to o} - 2 ,$$

where p_1 is the pressure amplitude of the fundamental, p_2 is the
pressure amplitude of the second harmonic, and x is progagation
distance[1,4,6]. A method which determines these quantities has
the potential for yielding B/A for optically opaque media and for
in vivo preparations.

Values of B/A have been obtained by measuring the harmonic
content of pulses of sound at various distances from the source
(3 MHz fundamental) and for varying concentrations in water of
several biological macromolecules of interest[5]. It has been found
that B/A appears to increase nearly linearly with increasing concentration of proteins and to exhibit little dependence upon molecular
weight (in the range 10^2 to 10^6 Daltons). These data suggest that
the nonlinearity parameter increases with decreasing intersolute
particle spacing. Thus it is clear that biological media exhibit
significant nonlinear ultrasonic propagation features which must be
studied in detail for deeper understanding leading to more sophisti-
cated diagnostic and therapeutic procedures.

REFERENCES

1.   R.T. Beyer and S.V. Letcher, in "Physical Ultrasonics", Academic
       Press, New York (1969), pp. 202-224.
2.   L.E. Kinsler and A.R. Frey, in "Fundamentals of Acoustics",
       John Wiley, New York (1962), 2nd ed., pp. 108-113.
3.   W.J. Fry and F. Dunn, Ultrasound: analysis and experimental
       methods in biological research, in "Physical Techniques in
       Biological Research", W.L. Nastuk, ed., Academic Press,
       New York (1962), Vol. 4, Ch. 6, pp. 261-394.
4.   E. Fubni-Ghiron, Anomalie nella propagazione di onde acustiche
       di grande ampiezza, Alta Frequenza 4:530-581 (1935).
5.   W.K. Law, L.A. Frizzell and F. Dunn, Ultrasonic determination
       of the nonlinearity parameter B/A for biological media,
       J. Acoust. Soc. Am. 69:4 (1981).
6.   L. Adler and E.A. Hiedmann, Determination of the nonlinearity
       parameter B/A for water and m-xylene, J. Acoust. Soc. Am.
       34:410-411 (1962).

ACKNOWLEDGEMENT

     This work was supported by the NSF and the NIH.

PROPAGATION OF ULTRASOUND IN SOLUTIONS OF BIOLOGICAL SUBSTANCES

A.P. Sarvazyan

Institute of Biological Physics
Academy of Sciences of the USSR
Pushchino (Moscow Region) 142292, USSR

The values of ultrasound velocity and absorption coefficient in solutions are defined by different molecular interactions. There is a large amount of literature on the investigation of molecular characteristics of solutions of biological substances by ultrasonic measurements. The dominant part of this paper is devoted to the measurements of the frequency dependences of ultrasound absorption and the investigation of fast relaxation processes. Substantially fewer works are related to the study of solutions by ultrasound velocity measurements. But such a proportion is a result of the absence of adequate velocity measurement methods and not due to the fact that the absorption coefficient is more informative than the velocity of ultrasound about the characteristics of a solution.

The purpose of this short review is to show the relationships between acoustic characterstics of biological solutions and their molecular properties, with emphasis on the ultrasound velocity. There are two reasons for such intentions:

(a) The possibilities of ultrasound velocity measurements in the investigation of biological substances in solutions are much less known, and

(b) The value of ultrasound velocity reflects to a greater extent the molecular characteristics of solutions of biological substances than absorption.

ABSORPTION OF ULTRASOUND

    The value of ultrasound absorption in a liquid characterizes
losses in the propagating wave energy, due to shear and bulk viscosi-
ties, thermoconductivity, and different relaxation processes occurring
during compression and decompression cycles in the sound field. The
latter is the main factor of the absorption of ultrasound in solutions
of most biological substances, especially those with high molecular
weight.

    The main relaxation processes which can occur in biological
solutions are perturbations of proton transfer and ion binding
processes, conformational equilibria, hydration and hydrogen bonding
equilibria. Relaxation processes can be detected by the measurement
of the frequency dependence either of the velocity or the absorption
of ultrasonic waves. But because of the absence of precise methods
of ultrasound velocity measurement within a wide enough frequency
range, only absorption measurements are used for such studies.
Aqueous solutions of biopolymers, the most important being proteins
and nucleic acids, at neutral pH show a wide spectrum of relaxation
processes which are attributed mainly to the segmental motion of the
backbone and side groups of polymer molecules. This spectrum is
very similar for all biopolymers and even for many synthetic polymers.
The dependence of ultrasound absorption in solutions of biopolymers
on the frequency, if drawn in double-logarithmic scale, is represented
by a straight line within nearly all the experimentally accessible
frequency range[1].

    Ultrasound absorption in solutions of proteins shows maxima in
both alkaline and acid regions due to proton transfer processes
involving dissociation of ionizable aminoacid residues. This process
in proteins and aminoacids is the most often investigated relaxation
phenomenon in solutions of biological substances[2,3]. A quantitative,
detailed description of thermodynamic and kinetic characteristics
of this process is obtained. There are some other successful applications of ultrasound absorption measurements in solutions of
biological substances for relaxation studies, e.g. for investigation
of stacking association and sin-anti transition of nucleic bases[4,
5,6]. But as a whole, ultrasonic absorption spectroscopy has not
contributed much of significance to molecular biology.

VELOCITY OF ULTRASOUND

    The systematic investigation of the relationship of ultrasound
velocity in solutions of biological substances to their molecular
characteristics has started only within the last decade, following
the appearance of adequate methods of measurement having the necessary
precision (about 10^{-6}) and allowing for measurements in small volumes
of liquids (0.1-1.0 ml)[7]. But the origin of these investigations

is in the early works of Passinsky[8], Jacobson[9], Shiio[10], Goto and Isemura[11], Dunn and Kessler[12] and other authors.

The difference between ultrasound velocities in aqueous solutions and in pure water is a result of three main contributions:

(a) changes in compressibility and density of the solvent due to the hydration process,

(b) intrinsic compressibility and density of the solute, and

(c) relaxational compressibility if some relaxation process is present.

These contributions are schematically shown in Fig. 1. The most important contribution in the case of solutions of low molecular substances is that of hydration. The main approach to the investigation of the hydration of complex biological molecules and the corresponding changes in ultrasound velocity is the comparative analysis of acoustical characteristics of solutions containing certain sequences of molecules[13,14]. The approach is based on the fact that the value of the ultrasound velocity increment in an aqueous solution being equal to the relative change in velocity over concentration of the solute $A=U/U_o.c$ is an additive function of the contributions of different parts of the hydration sphere of the solvent molecule, providing these parts do not interact[13].

The highly hydrated sites of solute molecules are charged groups. Changes in ultrasound velocity in a solution due to the appearance and disappearance of charged groups can be directly measured by pH

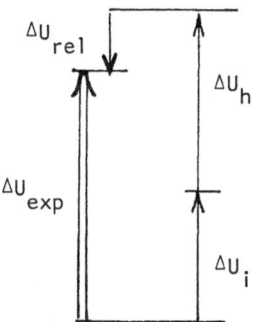

Fig. 1. Experimental value of the increment of ultrasound velocity represented as a sum of three contributions due to:
(a) intrinsic compressibility of solute molecules (ΔU_i),
(b) hydration (ΔU_h), and
(c) relaxation compressibility (ΔU_{rel}).

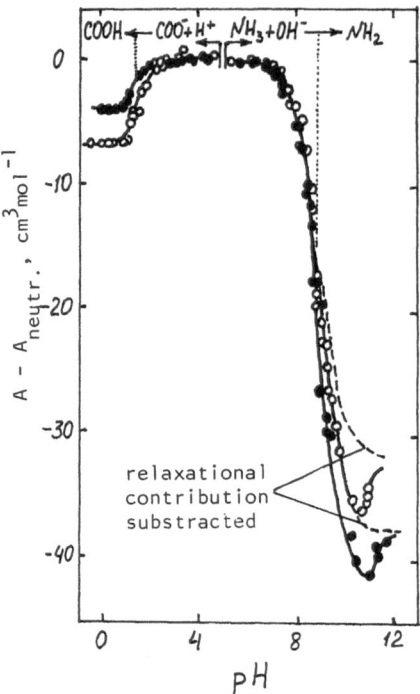

Fig. 2. Ultrasonic titration curves for glycine and adenine.

titration of these groups. Fig. 2. presents an example of such
titration: the dependences of ultrasound velocity increment A for
solutions of glycine and alanine on pH. Such dependences allow one
to estimate quantitatively the hydration effect of the dissociation
of an atomic group as well as the influence of the neighboring groups
on that hydration. It can be seen, for example, that the influence
of the aliphatic radical of alanine is opposite for the hydration of
positive and negative charges on the molecule. (In Fig. 2. compare
titration curves for glycine and alanine in acidic and alkaline
regions.) The relaxational contribution to ultrasound velocity increment can be seen on the titration curves of Fig. 2. in the alkaline
region. The contribution calculated from ultrasound absorption
measurements is subtracted from the titration curve and the dotted
lines show this difference, the latter being purely a hydrational
contribution. For solutions of proteins it was shown that the
relaxational contribution to ultrasound velocity increment is usually
small[15]. The contribution of intrinsic compressibility to ultrasound velocity increment can be neglected for small molecules in
solutions, but it becomes significant for globular proteins and
molecular complexes. Fig. 3. presents a scale of parameter A for
the number of proteins. Fibrillar proteins, being highly hydrated,
are in the upper part of the scale. Globular proteins, for which
the surfaces accessible to the solvent are much smaller, are placed

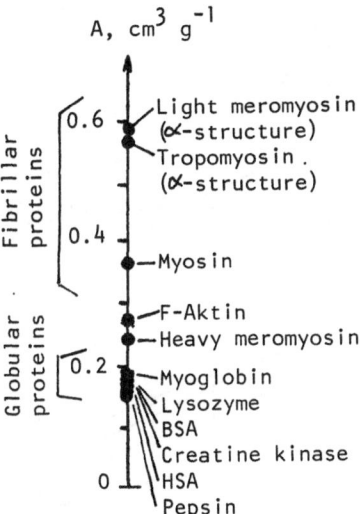

Fig. 3. Scale of ultrasound velocity increments for proteins

much lower on the scale. It was shown that the position of globular proteins on such a scale depends on the ratio of the surface of the protein globule to its volume and the contribution of its intrinsic compressibility is comparable to the hydrational contribution[14]. The value of the compressibility coefficient of a globule estimated from ultrasound velocity measurements is equal to:

$$(15\pm2) \cdot 10^{-12} m^2 \cdot N^{-1} \text{ (14)}.$$

Measurements of ultrasound velocity in suspensions of phospholipid bilayer vesicles as a function of temperature and concentration of salt allowed us to separate the hydration contribution of the vesicules to the parameter A, and to estimate the intrinsic compressibility of the hydrophobic part of the phospholipid bilayer. At room temperature and in a saltless solution that compressibility is:

$$(58.7\pm5.9) \cdot 10^{-11} m^2 \cdot N^{-1} \text{ (16)}.$$

Ultrasound velocity increment A of a solution of biological molecules is very sensitive to the nature of their hydrated sites. Fig. 4. shows the temperature dependences of velocity increment for NaCl, glycine and some aminoacid side chains. The value of A for side chains is obtained by substracting a value of glycine from that of a corresponding aminoacid. It can be seen that both the absolute value of A as well as its temperature slope are different for presented atomic groups.

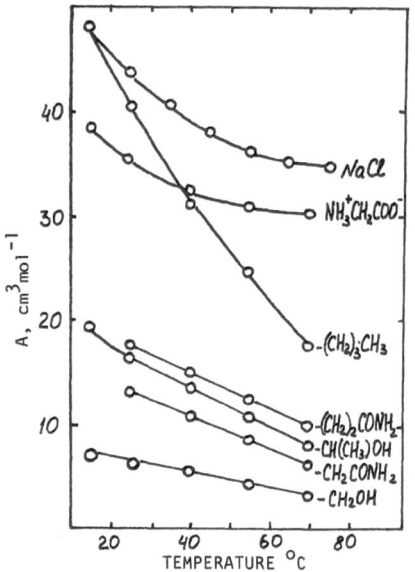

Fig. 4. Temperature dependences of ultrasound velocity increments
         for different molecules and atomic groups.

     An analysis of such dependences allows one to estimate the
relationship between ultrasound velocity increments of biological
molecules and their chemical structure.

     Many important processes in solutions of biopolymers such as
the formation of macromolecular complexes and conformational transitions are reflected in the value of ultrasound velocity. If a
process is accompanied by rearrangement of hydrophobic and charged
groups exposed to the solvent, or by changes in intrinsic compressibility, then it is possible to register such process by ultrasound
velocity measurements. An example of a conformational transition in
a solution of a biopolymer resulting in ultrasound velocity changes
is presented in Fig. r. Heat denaturation of a globular protein

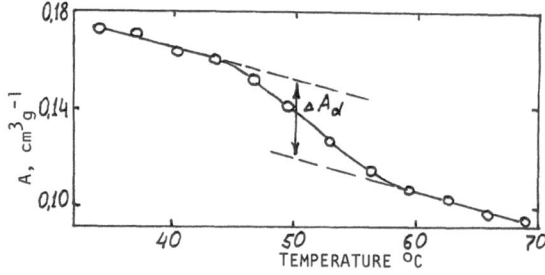

Fig. 5. Heat denaturation of α-chymotrypsinogen

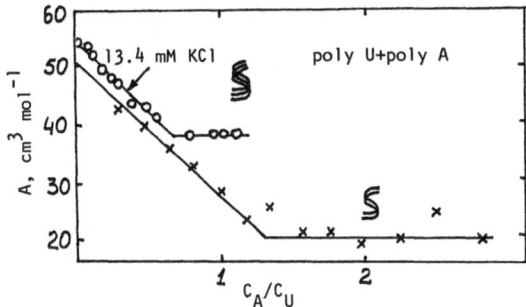

Fig. 6. Conformational transitions in solutions of polynucleotides

α-chymotrypsinogen leads to a change of ultrasound velocity increment A_d, which can be explained by 25-30% increase of its intrinsic compressibility. An example of ultrasound velocity changes due to the formation of macromolecular complexes is presented in Fig. 6., showing the dependence of parameter A in the mixed solution of polyadenine and polyuridine on the ratio of their concentrations[18]. At high ionic strength of the solution and increasing the ratio poly A : poly U from 0 to 0.5, triple helix 2 (poly A) poly U is formed. At lower ionic strength, double helix poly A poly U is formed.

Summarizing this part of the present brief review it can be stated that ultrasound velocity measurements may become an effective tool in the solution of problems of molecular biology.

REFERENCES

1. R.L. Johnston, S.A. Goss, V. Maynard, J.K. Brady, L.A. Frizzell, W.D. O'Brien, Jr. and F. Dunn, in "Ultrasonic Tissue Characterization II", M. Linzer, ed., NBS Special publication 25, Washington (1979), p. 20.
2. R.D. White and L.I. Slutsky, Biopolymers 11:1973 (1972).
3. H. Inoui, J. Sci. Hiroshima Univ. Ser. A-II 34:17 (1970).
4. D. Proshke and F. Eggers, Eur. J. Biochem. 26:490 (1972).
5. L.M. Rhodes and P.R. Shimmel, Biochemistry 10:4426 (1971).
6. P.R. Hemmes, L. Oppenheimer and F. Jordan, J. Am. Chem. Soc. 96:6023 (1974).
7. A.P. Sarvazyan, in "Abstracts of the Tenth International Congress on Acoustics", F-10,2, Sydney (1980).
8. A.G. Passinsky, J. Phys. Chem. (Rus.) 10:606 (1938).
9. B. Jacobson, Archiv für Kemi 2(11):177 (1950).
10. H. Shiido, J. Am. Chem. Soc. 80:70 (1958).
11. S. Goto and T. Isemura, Bull. Chem. Soc. Japan 37(11):1697 (1964).
12. L.W. Kessler and F. Dunn, J. Phys. Chem. 73:4256 (1969).

13. A.P. Sarvazyan, V.A. Buckin and P. Hemmes, J. Phys. Chem 84:629
    (1980).
14. A.P. Sarvazyan and D.P. Kharakoz, in "Molecular and Cellular
    Biophysics", Nauka, Moscow (1977), p. 93.
15. A.P. Sarvazyan and P. Hemmes, Biopolymers 18:3015 (1979).
16. V.A. Buckin, A.P. Sarvazyan and V.I. Passechnic, Biophysica
    (Rus.) 24:61 (1979).
17. D.P. Kharakoz and A.P. Sarvazyan, Studia Biophyica 79:179 (1980).
18. V.A. Buckin and A.P. Sarvazyan, Studia Biophysica 79:77 (1980).

ADVANCED METHODS FOR MEASURING SHEAR WAVE VELOCITY

IN BIOLOGICAL SUBSTANCES

S. Sajauskas and L. Juozoniene

Ultrasonic Laboratory
of the Polytechnical Institute
of Antanas Sniechkus,
Kaunas, USSR.

The measurement of shear wave velocity in biological tissues delivers much information on the tissue state and its structure. It may be used in diagnosis of different tumors. Such measurements involve some difficulties; for instance a transducer is necessary, which radiates pure shear waves into the tissue and does not generate longitudinal wave components. The possibly excited longitudinal waves, the attenuation of which is essentially lower than that of shear waves, may disturb the shear wave measurements, and for this reason longitudinal waves are highly undesirable.

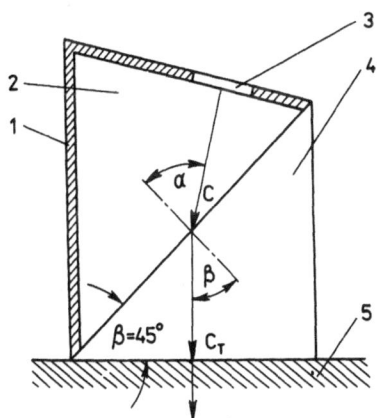

Fig. 1. The shear wave transducer construction:
1 - liquid prism; 2 - solid prism; 3 - piezoelectric transducer; 4 - tissue.

In the following, new techniques of measuring with shear waves which are free of longitudinal components will be investigated. The new transducer is shown in Fig. 1.

The probe consists of a piezoelectric transducer, a liquid prism with an angle α and a solid prism with the angle $\beta = 45^\circ$. If the following conditions are fulfilled:

$$\alpha = \text{arc sin} \frac{C}{\sqrt{2}\ C_T} \quad ,$$

$$\frac{\rho_1}{\rho_2} = \frac{C_T}{C} \sqrt{2 - \left(\frac{C}{C_T}\right)^2}$$

$$0 < \frac{C}{C_T} < \sqrt{2} \tag{1}$$

where C is the sound velocity in the liquid,
    C_T is the shear wave velocity in the solid prism,
    ρ_1 is the liquid density, and
    ρ_2 is the density of the solid prism,

a total reflection of the longitudinal waves occurs. Longitudinal waves do not appear in the solid prism because the transmission coefficient is zero at the angle $\beta = 45^\circ$. Pure shear waves are then excited in the solid prism by a mode conversion and are transmitted perpendicular to the tissue. By this technique no longitudinal waves occur in the transmission from the prism into the tissue.

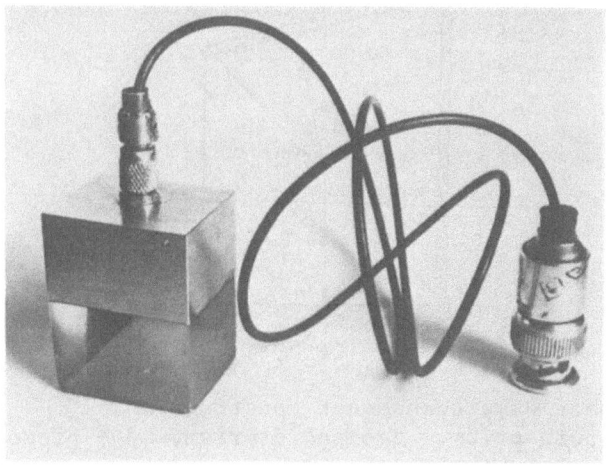

Fig. 2.   2 MHz shear wave probe.

A 2 MHz probe, which generates shear waves, is shown in Fig. 2. The probe consists of a prism with an angle of $\alpha = 52°20$, made from butylalcohol (C = 1265 m/s at $T° = 20°C$, $\rho_1 = 0.804$ g/cm^3) and a prism with an angle of $\beta = 45°$, made from polystyrene (C = 1120 m/s at $T° = 20°C$, $\rho_1 = 1.06$ g/cm^3).

An essential disadvantage is the necessity for a rigid contact between the probe and the specimen, using a shear wave transducer. This fact is very unfortunate for the measurement of biological materials. Therefore more suitable techniques are those based on the shear wave generation actually in the specimen to be examined.

The biological specimen was contained in a triangular cuvette (Fig. 3.). Then the incident angle α of the wave was changed to the angle α_T, at which the shear waves, transmitted into the specimen, were perpendicular to the back wall of the cuvette. In this case the shear waves, reflected from the back wall, were transformed into longitudinal waves, which can be picked up with the same transducer. This means the angle α_T is measured. The shear wave velocity may be calculated by the following formula:

$$C_T = C \frac{\sin \beta}{\sin \alpha_T} , \tag{2}$$

where β is the angle of cuvette.

The longitudinal waves in the specimen were the main source of error, which may disturb the shear wave measurements because of multiple reflections. To exclude these errors an immersion medium with a very slow sound velocity and an angle as high as possible should be chosen.

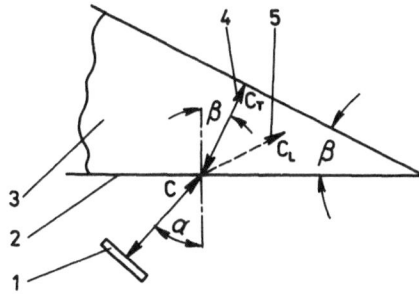

Fig. 3. Puls-technique of shear wave measurements:
1 - piezoelectric transducer; 2 - triangular cuvette;
3 - specimen; 4 - shear waves; 5 - longitudinal waves.

Thereby the following conditions must be fulfilled:

$$C < C_L \sin \alpha_T \quad ,$$

$$\beta < \text{arc} \sin \frac{C_T}{C_L} \quad , \tag{3}$$

where C_L is the velocity of longitudinal waves in the specimen to be examined.

In this case a total reflection of longitudinal waves occurs and pure shear wave measurements can be carried out in the tissue specimen.

To fulfil the condition (3) a fluid fluorcarbon compound was used, with a very slow sound velocity of $C = 420$ m/s at $T^0 = 20^0 C$.

The shear wave measurements in gel-type biological materials were carried out easily in a convenient rectangular cuvette (Fig. 4.).

If the sound velocity is so low that the measurements were carried out without longitudinal waves, then no longitudinal waves were excited in the specimen either.

In this case one can reach a relatively high accuracy of measurements, limited by the field diffraction effects, the accuracy of the angle α_T and the backscattering effects.

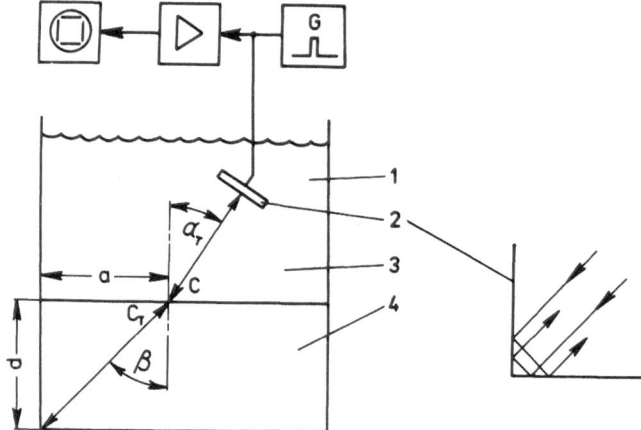

Fig. 4. Puls-technique of shear wave measurements in geltype bio-
         logical materials: 1 - immersion medium; 2 - piezoelectric
         transducer; 3 - rectangular cuvette; 4 - gel-type material.
         The wave reflection at the rightangle is shown separately.

AN ULTRASONIC MOVEMENT DETECTOR FOR TEST ANIMALS:

REGISTRATION METHOD AND EFFECTS OF AIRBORNE ULTRASOUND

ON ANIMAL BEHAVIOR

E. Rosenfeld, W.D. Grosse*, S. Berndt* and J. Schuh*

Institute of Applied Biophysics
*Division of Biological Sciences
Department of Zoology,
Martin Luther University, Halle, GDR

INTRODUCTION

For many behavioral-biological problems it is necessary to have definite information on the motoric activity of the test animals. In contrast to classic methods such as the exercise wheel or the rocking cage, much importance has recently been attached in particular to contact free techniques such as the capacitor or coil field methods.

In this context we want to report on an ultrasonic device, which is suitable for registering the motoric activity of test animals of different sizes[1].

This device has been in the test stage for the past year and a half. During this time we have been working particularly on the question of the extent to which the methodically inflicted stress on the test animal is increased due to the use of ultrasound.

METHOD

The measuring system works on the ultrasound Doppler principle. Transmitter and receiver transducers are fitted onto the outside of the test animals' cage. The sonic transducer works on a frequency of 42 KHz. The animals act as sonic reflectors, or scatterers.

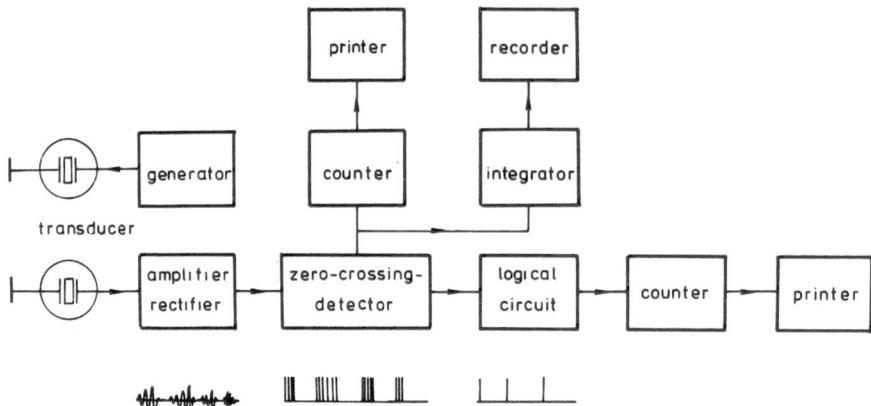

Fig. 1. Block diagram of the movement detector

The signals received are amplified and rectified and then converted into norm pulses using a zero crossing detector. The number
of impulses per time unit gives a scale for the distance covered in
this time and thus for the motoric activity. The impulses are counted
and the results are printed out. An integration of the impulse
sequence for the purpose of analogous registering occurs simultaneously (Fig. 1.).

However, apart from the amount of movement it is also useful to
have an evaluation of the extent of movement for some measurement
problems. This unit essentially consists of a counter, connected to
the zero-crossing-detector, which is set back to zero if the pause
between two impulses oversteps a certain time-limit. In this way
the number of impulses per burst corresponds to the extent of that
movement (idealized case). Since the different counter outputs allow
the choice of specific burst lengths for recording, the motoric
activity can be registered depending on the extent (e.g. type) of
the movements of the animal (Fig. 1., lower branch).

RESULTS AND DISCUSSION

The method is tried out next on several different types of test
animals to examine its usage on different sized animals. Fig. 2.
shows the activity of a rabbit dependent on the time of day. The
animal was kept in a normal wire cage and the light was controlled
using an instant light-dark change between 6 a.m. and 6 p.m. The
ultrasound method can be compared with a second method, the rocking
cage (applied simultaneously) and a reference measurement, carried
out with the rocking cage without the sonic influence and using
another animal. The two curves in the upper diagram correspond well
and also give a good representation of the "classic" curve below.

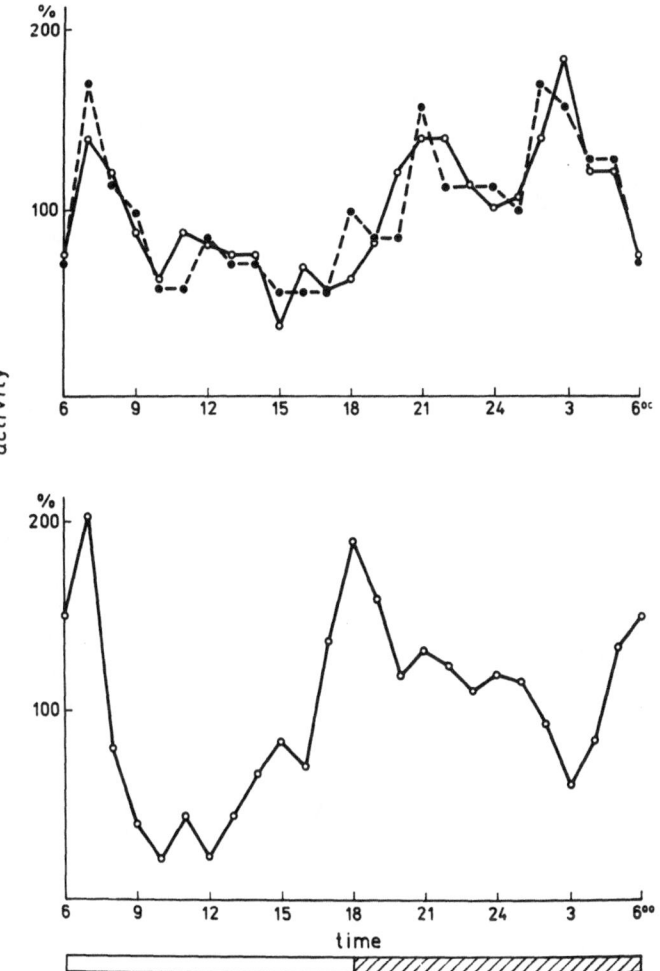

Fig. 2.   Locomotor activity of rabbit (Oryctolagus cuniculus (L.) f.
          domestica, race "Weisse Neuseeländer"):
          (a) ultrasound registration (open circle, rocking cage
          (solid circle)); (b) rocking cage without ultrasound
          according to (2).

    In Fig. 3. the motoric activity of mice is demonstrated. The
ultrasonic method is shown in comparison with the coil field method.

    The ultrasonic method can also be used on animals as small as
flies. The diagram in Fig. 4. shows the pattern of activity of
approximately forty flies. The ultrasound curve can be compared with
a light barrier curve, taken simultaneously and a light barrier
registering without ultrasound. All curves show the typical pattern
for animals active under light conditions.

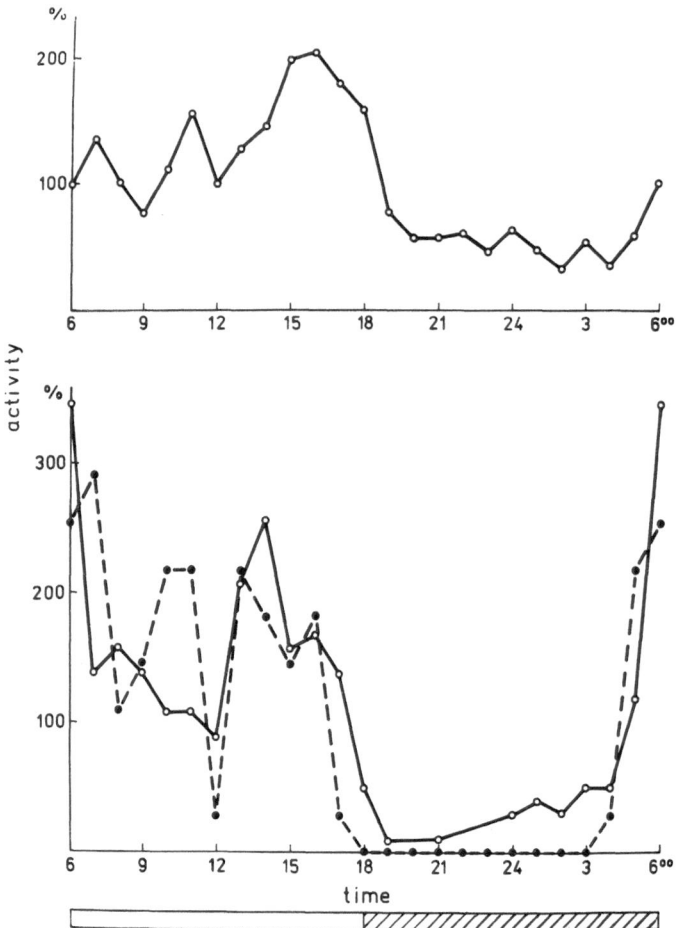

Fig. 3. Motoric activity of white mice (ICR–Line "Schönwalde"):
(a) ultrasound registration; (b) coil field method
(ANIMEX, LKB).

All ultrasound measurement results shown were made by registering
over a period of a few days. For routine usage of this method in
the laboratory the question of absence of side-effects is of particular interest. The diagrams presented in Figs. 1. to 4. give no
evidence of any significant influence on the animal behaviour through
the use of ultrasound.

In the following, results from ultrasound experiments carried
out over longer periods of time are presented. The investigations
were carried out on golden hamsters and Dsungarian hamsters over a
period of thirty days. The light conditions were the same as
described above. Fig. 5. demonstrates the activity patterns from
two series (J_1 and J_2) of experiments on golden hamsters. The ultra-

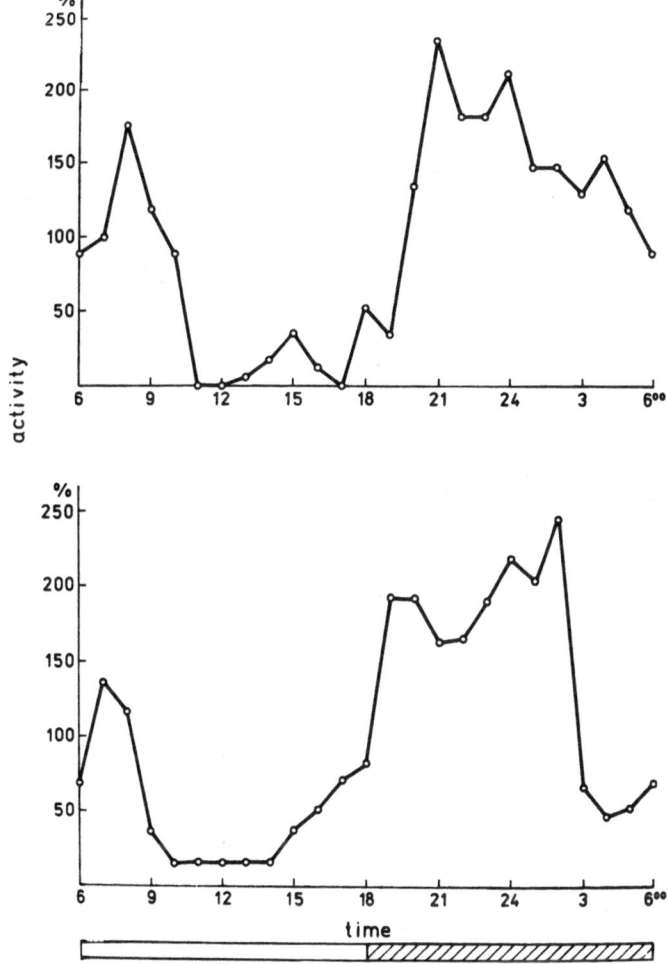

Fig. 4.   Motoric activity of flies (Calliphora erythrocephala Meig.);
          (a) ultrasound registration;   (b) light barrier registration,
          simultaneous with ultrasound (solid circles), without ultra-
          sound influence (open circles).

sound results were compared with light barrier results, registered
without the influence of ultrasound. Both were taken over a period
of ten days. The thick curve represents the average value and the
two thin ones show the 95%-confidence-interval. The comparison
between both methods shows that in all cases the typical activity of
nocturnal animals is registered. The ultrasound curves, however,
have additional modulations. These peaks can be traced to smaller
movements such as behavioral cleaning and similar movements. These
movements are not registered by the light barrier method, because
here only clear locomotion is registered.

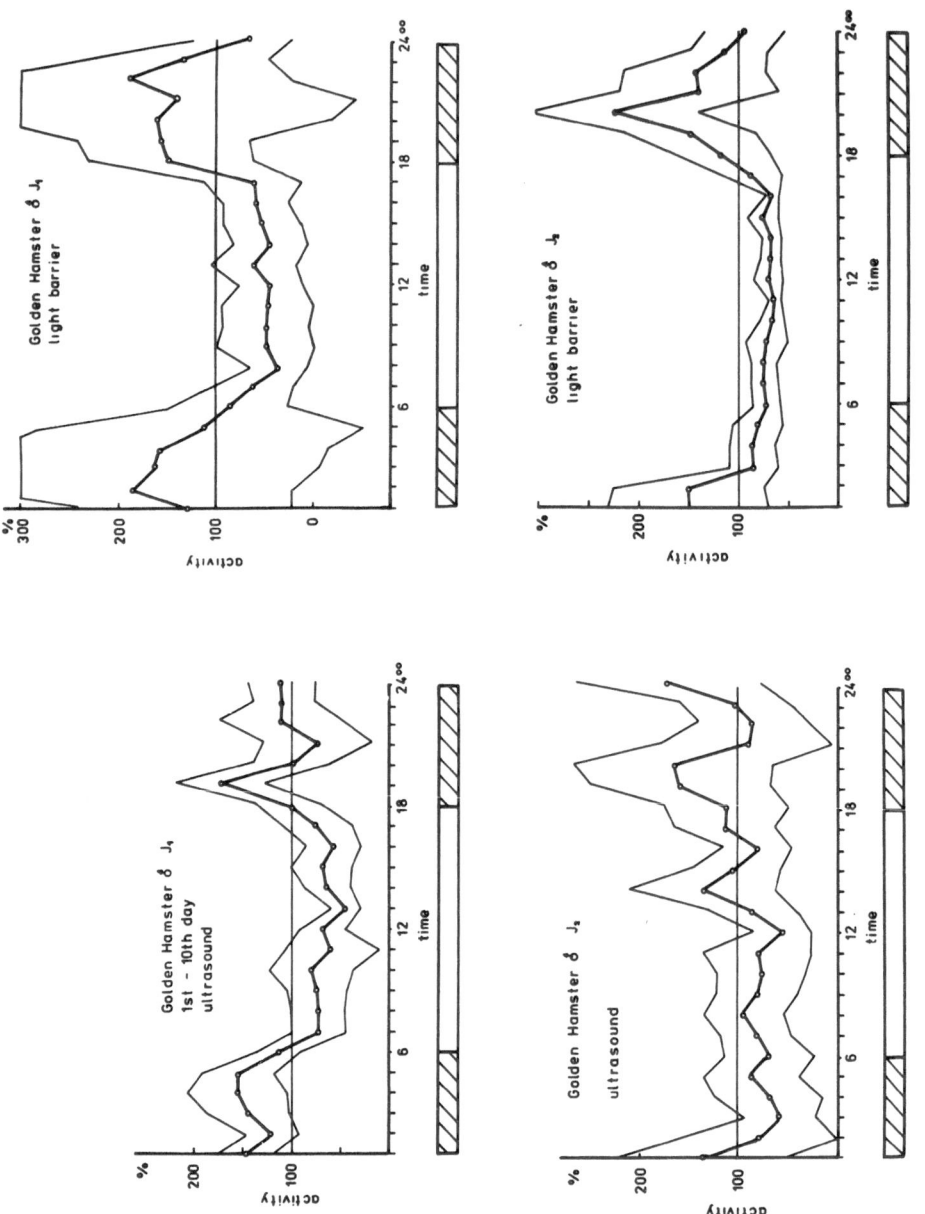

Fig. 5. Comparison between ultrasound and light barrier registration of the motoric activity

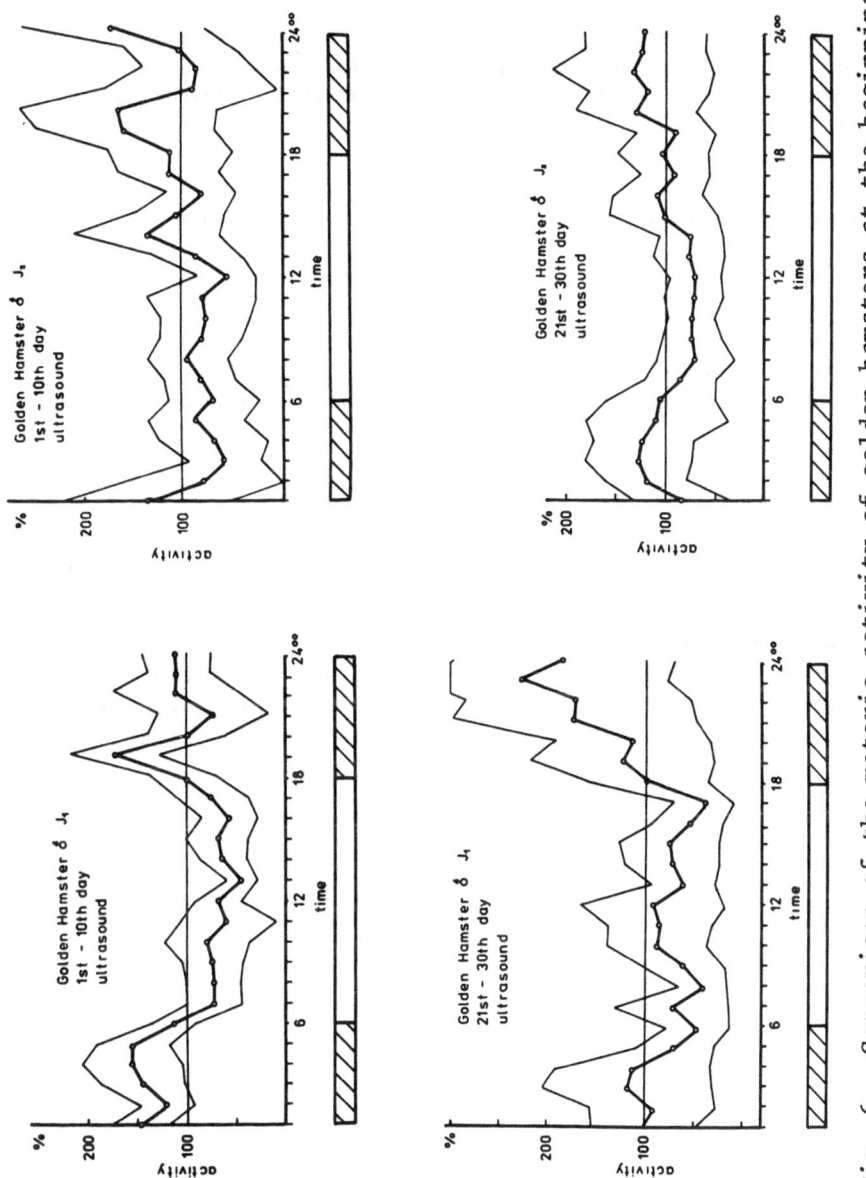

Fig. 6. Comparison of the motoric activity of golden hamsters at the beginning and at the end of the experimental period.

The comaprison of the activity curves at the beginning and at the end of the experiment period shows that there is no significant difference between both registrations (Fig. 6.). This means that on the basis of activity measurements an influence of airborne ultrasound on golden hamsters cannot be established.

In contrast to golden hamsters, preliminary experiments on Dsungarian hamsters point to different results. These animals show a certain ultrasonic sensitivity. The normal rhythm of activity is disturbed after two or three days in the sonicated cage. Movements are registered then during the true rest period too. The animal shows signs of stress in its behavior which is, however, reversible. After the cessation of sonication the normal activity patterns appear again.

In conclusion it can be established that the ultrasound movement detector can be of importance to biologists in its usage as a new contact free registering method for the motoric activity of test animals. The suitability of the method should, however, be examined in every case, depending on the type of test animal used.

REFERENCES

1. E. Rosenfeld, W.R. Grosse, J. Schuh and R. Millner, Ein Ultraschallverfahren zur Registrierung der motorischen Aktivität von Versuchstieren, Z. Versuchstierk. 22:89 (1980).
2. J. Schuh, Beitrag zur Analyse circadianer rhythmenphysiologischer Funktionen und Verhaltensgrössen bei Hauskaninchen Oryctolagus cuniculus (L.), f. domestica, Thesis Halle (1977).

INDEX